OVER- PRESCRIBING MADNESS

What's driving Australia's mental illness epidemic?

DR MARTIN WHITELY

Published by:
Wilkinson Publishing Pty Ltd
ACN 006 042 173

PO Box 24135, Melbourne, Victoria, Australia 3001
Ph: 03 9654 5446
www.wilkinsonpublishing.com.au

A catalogue record for this
book is available from the
National Library of Australia

Planned date of publication: 02-2021
Title: Overprescribing Madness
ISBN(s): 9781925927535: Paperback

Design by Spike Creative Pty Ltd
Ph: (03) 9427 9500
spikecreative.com.au

Printed and bound in Australia by Griffin Press, part of Ovato

About the author

Dr Martin Whitely is a mental health researcher, author, former mental health consumer advocate, teacher, and Member of the West Australian Parliament. His research interests include regulatory capture of mental health policy and practice, especially in relation to the safe use of drugs for ADHD and depression.

Martin is a Research Fellow at the John Curtin Institute of Public Policy at Curtin University and has led award winning research demonstrating that the youngest children in a classroom both in Western Australia and globally are much more likely than their older classmates to be 'medicated' for ADHD.

After leaving politics Martin worked as a mental health consumer advocate, supporting 'patients' during psychiatric consultations. Martin was struck by the enormous variation in the quality of psychiatric practice: "Some psychiatrists were wonderful. They treated the consumer as an equal partner. However, others had absolutely no empathy. Worse still, some were bullies."

Martin's first book *Speed Up and Sit Still – the controversies of ADHD diagnosis and treatment* was published in 2010 (UWA Publishing). In 2014 he completed his PhD thesis titled *Attention Deficit Hyperactivity Disorder (ADHD) Policy, Practice and Regulatory Capture in Australia 1992–2012*. In his thesis Martin investigated the relationship between Australian ADHD child prescribing rates and 'regulatory capture' of ADHD policy and practice nationally, and in WA and New South Wales.

Martin is the publisher and editor of Psychwatch Australia.

Contents

Madness in the Age of COVID-19

This book was finished in the middle of the COVID-19 pandemic. So far Australia has been admirably successful in limiting viral infections and deaths. But this achievement has come at a considerable cost. Shutdowns, particularly in the hospitality, retail and tourist industries, have cost jobs and caused business failures. For many Australians social isolation has meant just that – isolation and loneliness.

Prominent Australian psychiatrists Professors Ian Hickie and Patrick McGorry, along with President of the Australian Medical Association, Dr Tony Bartone, predicted that these factors may result in a spike in suicides.[1] In May 2020 the Hickie-led *Brain and Mind Centre* published modelling that predicted the COVID-19 crisis would lead to a 25% jump in the suicide rate if unemployment surges 11%. McGorry predicted the deaths and damage caused by mental illness would overshadow those caused by COVID-19. Both McGorry and Hickie called on the Commonwealth and state governments to spend hundreds of millions more funding mental health interventions.[2]

They may be right. The despair caused by unemployment, financial hardship and loneliness may well lead to an increase in suicides that dwarfs the loss of life in Australia from COVID-19. However, is it appropriate to pour hundreds of millions of dollars into mental health services as the Professors demand?

Their call for extra mental health funding would be entirely logical if the care on offer actually helped people distressed by unemployment, financial hardship and loneliness. But sadly, as is detailed in this book, the evidence is that far too often the mental health care on offer – including that promoted by Hickie and McGorry – does more harm than good.

The reality for most Australians seeking mental health help is a visit to the GP, a drug prescription – most often an antidepressant – and a bit of a chat about possible side effects if you are lucky. There is a role for drugs, but we are far too reliant on a quick diagnosis backed up by indiscriminate prescribing of pills that messily interfere with a patient's biochemistry without addressing their underlying problems.

The key to preventing suicides and despair caused by COVID-19 related loneliness, job and business losses is to tackle loneliness and protect jobs and businesses. It is a tragic irony that medicalising these problems by expanding mental health services may ultimately result in more suffering and even avoidable deaths.

If this seems far-fetched, consider Australia's recent history of suicide prevention among young Australians. As detailed in Chapter 5, in the late 2000s, debate raged about how we should best tackle the scourge of youth suicide. Despite US FDA warnings about a link between antidepressant use and suicidal thinking and behaviour in young people, prominent Australian suicide prevention organisations and experts – including Hickie and McGorry – encouraged young Australians to seek help, including treatment with antidepressants claiming this would decrease suffering and prevent suicide. Since 2009 – as I and others involved in the debate predicted[3] – Australia has seen rapidly rising rates of both antidepressant use and suicide among young Australians.

This is just one example of many of 21st century mental health interventions massively over-promising and under-delivering.

Unfortunately, given the current medicalised momentum of mental health policy in Australia, it appears likely we are about to see history repeat.

Chapter 1

Sicker, Sadder, Madder

Over the last decade, mental health – for so long ignored – has finally received attention. In laudable efforts to help destigmatise mental illness, sport stars, celebrities and politicians have publicly shared their personal battles with depression, bipolar disorder and a host of other mental health problems. Australian governments, both state and federal, have appointed specialist Mental Health Ministers, and significant resources are being committed to new and expanded mental health services.

To casual observers, it may appear that at last we are on track to a happier, mentally healthier tomorrow. However, appearances can be deceiving. The future direction of mental health outcomes in Australia is far from certain. Just about everybody involved in the debate agrees things need to change, but this is where the consensus ends.

There are at least three different approaches on offer. For the want of better names, I call them 'Americanisation', 'Preventive Psychiatry' and 'Recovery'. The Americanisation and Preventive Psychiatry approaches are two sides of the same coin. The former seeks to find new ways of identifying and treating mental illness. The latter seeks to spot tell-tale signs of emerging mental illness and prevent it before it occurs. Both promote growing rates of diagnosis and aggressive interventions. Both risk harm from imprecise labelling and unnecessary treatment. Both are very profitable for Big Pharma. In contrast, the consumer-led Recovery approach, when properly implemented, responds to the individual, not the diagnosis, has faith in their ability to get better, and respects the intent of 'first do no harm'.

While the direction we should take is contested, what is not in dispute is that, over the last decade, mental health has become a first-order issue. Media coverage and political focus on mental health have grown exponentially. However, the main outcome of this increased attention is that billions in taxpayer money has been spent on programs and treatments (primarily drugs), while Australians have on average become sicker, sadder and madder.

In 2018, over 1 in 6 Australians took at least one mental health-related drug[4], with roughly 1 in 8 taking an antidepressant, and since then prescribing rates have continued to rise.[5] Many Australians take multiple psychotropic medications. For example, many elderly people are prescribed antidepressants for anxiety or depression, along with antipsychotics to control agitation. Similarly, children prescribed amphetamines for Attention Deficit Hyperactivity Disorder (ADHD) are sometimes prescribed clonidine, or other downers (depressants) to help them sleep.

Our willingness to take pills and give them to our children, to ease perceived unhappiness, dysfunction and distress, is not new. Comparisons of 30 OECD countries in the year 2000, and again in 2015, both found that Australians were the second largest per-capita users of antidepressants. Only tiny Iceland (population 340,000), with its frozen, dark, miserable North Atlantic winters, had a higher per-capita antidepressant prescribing rate in either year.[6] Our propensity for using antidepressants is consistent with a 2017 World Health Organization (WHO) publication that reported that Australia was the equal second most depressed country in the world.[7]

These numbers may shock you but, according to reputable sources, including the Australian Bureau of Statistics, right now more than four million Australians are thought to be suffering from a mental illness. So, if you assume the drugs work, and you accept the official estimates of the prevalence of mental illness, it makes perfect sense that millions of Australians take psychiatric medication. However, the estimates of prevalence of mental illness are based on dodgy definitions of psychiatric disorders; and, for many patients, pills hurt far more than they help.

Medicalising Misery

At the heart of the problem is how we have come to define mental health and mental illness. Anything that causes us to be sad, stressed, anxious, or even bored is now regarded as a threat to our mental health, and therefore a potential source of mental illness. If you lose your job, are grieving a death or a relationship breakdown, or are experiencing any of life's inevitable vicissitudes, then it is very human to be deeply unhappy or anxious and some may even fleetingly consider ending it all. But we have come to regard these normal, although troubling, human reactions as compelling evidence of mental illness.

We have blindly followed the lead of American psychiatry, which has progressively medicalised normality. In effect, we have outsourced our definitions of mental illness to the country that spends the most per-capita on mental health but achieves appalling outcomes.[8]

While many Australians decry the effects that Hollywood, Coca-Cola, and McDonald's have on our culture, most are completely ignorant about the dominant role American psychiatry plays in contemporary Australia. They have no idea that we have let the Americans define sanity and madness for us. This outsourcing has a massive impact on millions of Australians and their families. It is hard to think of a more powerful example of cultural capture.

What is even more disturbing is that this corrosive Americanisation of Australian psychiatric practice is officially endorsed by our governments. In 2017, the Australian Commonwealth Government and all state and territory governments agreed that mental illness is defined as a 'clinically diagnosable disorder' that significantly interferes with a person's cognitive, emotional or social abilities.[9] Of course individual 'clinically diagnosable disorders' are defined in the American Psychiatric Association's *Diagnostic and Statistical Manual of Mental Disorders 5th edition* (DSM-5).

The main problem with DSM-5 based psychiatry is that normal human suffering and frailty is classified as disease. The complexity of human behaviour is reduced to a tick box list of behaviours, devoid of empathy for individual differences in disposition and circumstance. Misery is medicalised, and claims of massive unmet mental health need become the orthodoxy.

Estimating the prevalence of a psychiatric disorder usually involves using DSM-5 behavioural criteria and surveying a sample of the population (or their parents in the case of children) to identify if they display 'disordered' behaviours. These behaviours are then overlayed upon the diagnostic criteria of all psychiatric disorders to identify what proportion of the population would qualify for a diagnosis. Sometimes, more rigorous researchers try to determine if the degree of perceived dysfunction or impairment reaches the diagnostic threshold. Occasionally, they may ask questions about external factors, like recent trauma, that may contribute to behaviour.

Irrespective of how thorough a prevalence rate estimate is, it invariably exceeds the current rate of diagnosis, particularly for the more controversial psychiatric disorders. This happens for one simple reason. Most potential patients (or parents who have children who would qualify for a diagnosis) are too sensible to allow themselves (or their child) to be given a psychiatric label. For example, if properly informed about the subjective behavioural basis of the diagnosis, and the nature of the drugs used to treat it, few competent parents would allow their child to be labelled ADHD, and be given a daily amphetamine habit.

Nonetheless, very high estimates of the prevalence of mental illness are accepted by most decision makers, including governments, who fail to understand the significant limitations of these estimates. For example, the Australian Parliamentary website contains a webpage titled, *Mental Health in Australia: a quick guide.*[10]

Excerpt from Parliament of Australia Website
Mental Health in Australia: a quick guide[11]

- The Australian Bureau of Statistics (ABS) National Survey of Mental Health and Wellbeing (NSMHWB) [conducted in 2007] provides the most comprehensive (albeit dated) estimates for mental disorders in Australian adults both over their lifetime and in the preceding 12 months. The survey estimated that 45 per cent of Australians had experienced a mental disorder in their lifetime, with 20 per cent experiencing a mental disorder in the previous year.

- The most recent ABS National Health Survey estimated there were 4.8 million Australians (20.1%) [that identify as having] a mental or behavioural condition in 2017–18. This was an increase of 2.6 percentage points from 2014–15, mainly due to an increase in the number of people reporting anxiety-related conditions, depression, or feelings of depression.

- The Australian Child and Adolescent Survey of Mental Health and Wellbeing, conducted between June 2013 and April 2014 by the Department of Health, estimated that almost 14 per cent of young people aged 4 to 17 years (or 560,000 children) experienced a mental disorder in the 12 months before the survey.

These inflated figures are used to argue that mental illness is being left unrecognised and untreated with disastrous consequences and that governments must support universal mental health screening in schools and in the workplace.

Alarming figures about the cost to the economy of unrecognised and untreated mental illness are also frequently cited. For example, in October 2019 there was widespread media coverage of a draft Productivity Commission report that estimated that as many as one million Australians are going untreated for mental health conditions and these 'illnesses' are costing the economy $500 million every day.[12]

This represents well over 10% of Australia's GDP, yet, despite the astonishing size of the estimated cost, it and similar claims rarely get challenged. Instead it is assumed that massive economic benefits are available if we just address unmet mental health needs. This analysis and other similar claims are based on two flawed assumptions. The first is that we can accurately identify who needs help (without massive false positives) and the second is that the help available (primarily drugs) fixes the problem.

More is Less

In Australia we have come to believe as an article of faith that spending more on mental health interventions improves outcomes and has economic benefits. However, in the USA since 1987, rapidly rising rates of mental health interventions have been associated with massive increases in the proportion of Americans receiving government disability support payments for mental illness. This comes with an obvious opportunity cost to both the individual and the economy.[13]

Sometimes the drugs that are used to treat psychiatric disorders create new disorders that are managed with other drugs. Often the withdrawal effects from psychiatric drugs are worse than the initial problems they were supposed to treat. This iatrogenic suffering (harm caused by treatment) is often blamed on the patient's re-emerging mental illness, and doses are increased and/or new medications are added. The result is the patient gets locked into a vicious cycle of drugs creating harm, with more drugs added to address that harm; meanwhile medication sales soar and Big Pharma rakes in iatrogenic profits (profits caused by creating harm).

There is mounting evidence of harms caused by psychiatric drugs, particularly antipsychotics (diabetes, metabolic syndrome, heart attacks, brain atrophy), antidepressants (suicidality, falls and injuries, birth abnormalities), and stimulants (addiction, psychiatric disorders, growth retardation, cardiovascular disorders etc.) that increases the demands on non-psychiatric health and welfare services.

This suffering is avoidable. Governments, doctors, patients and their families need to resist the sugar rush temptation of relying on pharmaceutical quick fixes for complex mental health and social problems. Ironically, the increasing use of psychotropic drugs temporarily takes the political pressure off governments to provide more resource-intensive but safer, and in the long term more effective and less expensive, interventions. Governments must recognise the harm caused by the over-prescription of the psychotropic drugs that they often subsidise. Otherwise they will continue to misallocate resources to options that superficially appear to address mental health need at minimal cost.

I know from personal interactions that many Australian psychiatrists do not want to practice pharmaceutical psychiatry and are very reluctant to label patients and prescribe medications. They have told me they would like to focus on understanding each patient's unique circumstances and respond appropriately, rather than quickly identifying a psychiatric disorder and prescribing the matching drug.

Although they want to practice in a less invasive fashion, economic factors favour the 'pill for every ill' model that dominates current psychiatric practice.

In many developed nations, a diagnosis of a specific psychiatric disorder is required for a psychiatrist to receive payment from governments or health insurers. Many governments also heavily subsidise pharmaceutical interventions but provide only limited support for behavioural interventions. There is also overwhelming evidence of regulatory capture by pharmaceutical companies of government drug approval and subsidisation processes that reinforces the dominance of pseudo-scientific Biological Psychiatry.[14]

Another obstacle for achieving safe and effective psychiatric practice is the dominant role that non-expert mental health practitioners, particularly general practitioners, play in the delivery of mental health services. The vast majority of the prescribing of mental health drugs in Australia is done by non-psychiatrists, especially general practitioners.[15] In 2018/19 according to the Australian Government '86.3% of mental health-related prescriptions were prescribed by GPs; 7.7% prescribed by psychiatrists; 4.5% prescribed by non-psychiatrist specialists'.[16] So even if the Australian psychiatric profession miraculously got its act together overnight and only prescribed psychotropic drugs within genuinely evidence-based parameters, this would have minimal effect. Sadly, non-expert, dumbed down, cookbook, DSM-5 based Biological Psychiatry has become the dominant model of psychiatric care in Australia, and it is going to take a revolution to change that.

Australia is not an isolated case. In all countries that have followed America's lead, as each new edition of the DSM has expanded the definitions of mental illness – and narrowed the definitions of normal – psychiatric drug sales have soared. As detailed in Chapter 2, this has not occurred by accident. The American Psychiatric Association

(APA) and pharmaceutical manufacturers have increasingly developed a co-dependent relationship that has manifested in a shift in emphasis from talking therapies to drugs. The APA is effectively in partnership with Big Pharma. And Big Pharma, the senior partner, is not just big, it is huge and getting bigger, with very healthy profit margins. The pharmaceutical industry's total global revenue in 2018 was over US$1.2 trillion (US$1,200,000,000,000 – about the size of Australia's GDP) and has grown rapidly from US$390 billion in 2001.[17]

Of course, some Big Pharma products are lifesaving, and many other lives, including mine, have been improved because of access to safe, effective pharmaceutical treatments. But Big Pharma does not exist to help people. Its dominant aim is to maximise profits and share prices, and every action it takes should be viewed in that light. In recent years, multiple large pharmaceutical companies have incurred multi-billion dollar fines, primarily in the USA, for dishonestly marketing drugs.[18] These fines have occurred so frequently – with no obvious deterrent effect – that it is clear that Big Pharma see them as just another cost of doing business.

It is also becoming increasingly apparent that the evidence supporting the use of many psychotropic drugs, including antidepressants and antipsychotics, has been dishonestly influenced by Big Pharma and their hired help. While some patients benefit from their cautious and monitored use – psychotropic drugs are massively overprescribed, with emerging evidence of real harm, especially growing rates of youth self-harm and suicide.

There is no doubt that there are new challenges to our mental wellbeing. We have designed our suburbs, houses and society with too much concern for privacy and too little concern about loneliness. Increasing materialism, the loss of low-skill jobs, and the casualisation of the workforce, have also had an impact on our wellbeing. However, there has also been many changes for the better. Prejudices about gender, race, religion, sexual preferences etc. have diminished, making Australia a much more inclusive society.

The evidence suggests that taking prescription psychotropic drugs in such large and increasing numbers is not helping us face new challenges or embrace new opportunities. Surveys suggest that Australians are still a relatively content and functional people. However, they also suggest that we are slowly going backwards in terms of happiness[19], social isolation, rates of psychosis and in international comparisons of numeracy and literacy – the very problems these 'treatments' are supposed to address.

Not all the responsibility lies with doctors or the 'system'. Many patients demand pills. They want a quick fix and are not open to other options. If they are fully informed about the true benefits and risks of treatments (which very often they are not) then that is their choice.

Parents make these decisions on behalf of their children. Many are attracted by the promise of immediate improvement in behaviours and do not pay proper regard to the long-term effects of medication use. Some even seek out clinicians who will tell them what they want to hear and prescribe the drugs they want for their children.

Much of this prescribing is 'off label', i.e. for conditions and/or populations that it has not been approved for, even if this contravenes the manufacturer's recommendations or product warnings. Off label prescribing occurs so regularly that it has, in many cases, become the norm. It does not necessarily result in adverse outcomes; sometimes patients benefit. But off label prescribing is unregulated and outside safety parameters established through the licencing process.

This should not be acceptable. Psychiatric practice should be based on robust independent evidence. Yet, collectively, Australians seem determined to spend even more on dubious treatments and overhyped programs, sometimes to fix problems in part created by dubious treatments and overhyped programs.

Many of the factors driving this escalating madness are identical to those in other developed nations. However, the influence of some homegrown key thought leaders, who have dominated the debate about the future of service delivery in Australia, should not be underestimated. More salesmen than scientists, these mental health gurus/entrepreneurs have secured hundreds of millions in taxpayer funds for their pet programs. They have massively overpromised and under-delivered, and yet to date they have not been held to account.

Successive Commonwealth Governments have unquestioningly accepted the hype and rhetoric around these programs and failed to thoroughly evaluate their outcomes. Worse still, these Governments have failed to carry out one of their core functions – ensuring that medications are used within robust evidence-based safety and efficacy parameters – in these services and elsewhere.

Big Pharma and their paid associates are incredibly good at gaming the systems of drug regulation and subsidisation. They charm, bamboozle and manipulate hapless politicians and limp regulators by creating the illusion that their products are supported by robust science. They are so good at manipulating research as a marketing tool that we should stop expecting the regulatory system to protect our health and well-being.

We should also stop being shocked by stories of 93-year-olds in nursing homes being drugged into a stupor with life-shortening heavy doses of antipsychotics[20], or of 7-year-olds given amphetamines, antidepressants and antipsychotics and wanting to take their own lives[21]. We must change the system, or at least wake up to the fact that evidence-free psychiatric prescribing is normal.

The most damning example of this failure is the wholesale off label prescribing of antidepressants to children and adolescents, despite

FDA and TGA warnings that antidepressant use increases suicidality in young people. As detailed in Chapter 4, child, adolescent and young adult antidepressant prescribing rates have soared over the last decade, and so has the rate of suicide among young Australians. From July 2017 to June 2018, at least 101,174 Australians aged 0 to 17 years (1.8% of the total number) were prescribed an antidepressant, despite the fact that no antidepressant is approved for the treatment of paediatric depression.[22]

It is highly plausible that this failure of government to ensure evidence-based prescribing has contributed significantly to Australia's epidemic of youth suicide. Yet our political leaders have continued to seek advice from the same failed suicide prevention gurus who obstinately deny the possibility that antidepressant use maybe part of the problem. If insanity is doing the same thing over and over again and expecting different results, then clearly Australia's mental health system has gone barking mad.

Politics – Where is the conflict when you actually need it?

Many aspects of Australian public policy could benefit from a more bipartisan approach. However, mental health is suffering from a lack of competition between political parties. For most politicians, mental health is a mysterious issue, and the simple option of subsidising the quick application of diagnostic labels and prescription of pills has superficial appeal. In addition, when charismatic mental health entrepreneurs claim to have 21st century solutions, many politicians clearly think: Who am I to argue? But there are sound reasons why both the Right and the Left should be suspicious of the direction of Australian mental health policy and practice.

Conservatives should be concerned about overreach by Big Government interfering in the lives of citizens by applying a permanent disability model of mental illness that robs us of our individual autonomy and self-reliance. The Left should be concerned about the influence of Big Pharma corrupting our regulatory processes and selling us products that are bad for us and make us sicker and more reliant on their products. The Centre should be concerned about both. But there is effectively no competition of ideas regarding mental health among Australian politicians. The only competition appears to be squabbling about who can give our high-profile mental health entrepreneurs the most money for their pet projects.

Despite this bleak picture, there are some green shoots of hope. Done with genuine intent, the Recovery approach centres on developing a patient's own capabilities and resilience and is less reliant on pills. As opposed to the 'ongoing disability' or 'impending doom' assumptions inherent in the American and Preventive Psychiatry approaches, the Recovery model is more optimistic about the capacity for individuals to get better. Implemented properly, it supports mentally ill patients with housing, educational, employment and psychosocial support – building blocks for a happy future that cannot be replaced by drugs.

While the Recovery approach is more optimistic about human resilience, it is more realistic about the limits of psychiatry than either of the other approaches. The Americanisation approach is based on the unrealistic assumption that psychiatric science can accurately identify over 300 disorders. Preventive Psychiatry is based on the fanciful notion that mental illness can be reliably spotted before it happens.

Although many proponents of Preventive Psychiatry have appropriated the language of the Recovery movement, in reality their approach is often a barrier to recovery. They seek to extend the American Psychiatric Association's permanent disability model by adding new categories of impending disability to individuals perceived to have an elevated risk of being mentally ill.

Both the Americanisation and Preventive approaches are justified using pseudo-science. Both approaches are fundamentally narcissistic where practitioners pretend – or are deluded in thinking – that they know much more than they actually do. Both grossly exaggerate their capacity to help. Both ignore the Hippocratic obligation to first do no harm.

Thankfully there are many cautious psychiatrists who realise the limitations of their profession and diagnose and medicate with great care. They resist incentives from industry and the pressure from 'the system', and in some cases from patients and carers, to concentrate primarily on short term symptom management. Their professionalism in alliance with the consumer-led psychiatric Recovery movement offers some hope that fewer patients will be prevented from recovering by being labelled and numbed by 'medications' on the assumption that, without them, they are biochemically imbalanced.

Unfortunately, a significant real-world disadvantage for the Recovery model is that, while it is optimistic about patients' prospects, it offers a pessimistic outlook for the profitability of pharmaceutical companies. If history is any indicator of the future, this failure to generate massive profits could prove to be its fatal flaw.

The Lucky Country – Why so sad?

Australia should be a country in which it is relatively easy to be happy and feel safe, affluent and secure. Australia's five largest cities are all ranked in the 22 most liveable cities in the world.[23] We enjoy (or rather can enjoy) abundant sunshine, clean air, sensational beaches and open spaces, great food, longevity, a world-class universal access health-care system, robust democracy, rule of law, political and religious freedom, relative economic equity, and a high standard of living following 28 years of unbroken economic growth before the COVID-19 recession.[24]

Clearly these positives are not enough to make all of us 'relaxed and comfortable'. For some Australians, mental illness can be debilitating;

and for some, psychotropic drugs, when used judiciously, are helpful. However, Australia has extraordinarily high and rising rates of antidepressant and other mental health drug use, and the World Health Organization rates Australians as the world's second most depressed people.[25]

It's time to ask, are things really that miserable in the lucky country? It may be that these disturbing statistics have nothing to do with Australians being disproportionately mentally ill. Rather, it appears a combination of slick salesmanship, dishonest and incompetent medical practice (overlooked by timid regulators) and cultural, commercial, and political drivers now see Australians hooked on a cycle of over-diagnosis and over-medication.

This book is written in the hope that telling the warts and all truth about the madness driving Australian mental health policy and practice, may help sanity prevail. Some of the truth seems unbelievable, most of it is inconvenient; but we really are spending an awful lot of money, energy, time and enthusiasm, following very bad advice, and doing things that make us sicker, sadder and madder.

Chapter 2

All the way
with the APA

The American Psychiatric Association (APA) is the major
professional organisation of psychiatrists in the USA and is the
largest psychiatric organisation in the world, with approximately
38,000 mainly US members. The APA publishes the *Diagnostic
and Statistical Manual of Mental Disorders* (DSM), often referred
to as the 'Bible of Psychiatry'. The first edition of the DSM was
published in 1952. It detailed the diagnostic criteria for 106
psychiatric disorders. The latest edition, DSM-5 was published
in 2013, and details 312 disorders. For some disorders
(e.g. schizophrenia), the criteria involve unusual behaviours like
hallucinations or catatonia. For other disorders (e.g. ADHD), the
diagnostic criteria are normal behaviours (fidgeting, disliking
homework, playing loudly etc.) that are considered to be displayed
too often.

Americans spend the most per-capita on mental health interventions,
use the most psychotropic drugs[26], and have the highest rates of
diagnosed psychiatric disorders[27] on the planet. America remains the
home of ADHD child drugging, with about 1 in 10 children (aged 2-17)
ever having been diagnosed with ADHD[28] and millions of children
prescribed antidepressants and/or antipsychotics.[29] None of this appears
to be working. American teenagers perform very poorly on numeracy

and literacy tests.[30] The USA is tumbling down global happiness rankings[31], and the life expectancy of Americans is shortening[32].

The USA should hardly provide the model for enhancing the mental health of Australians. However, the domination of Australian psychiatric practice by the American Psychiatric Association (APA), through the *Diagnostic and Statistical Manual of Mental Disorders* (DSM), ensures that is exactly what happens. On key measures – psychiatric drug use, diagnosis rates, measures of national happiness[33], and suicide rates[34] – Australia is following America's lead. Our rates of child prescribing are considerably lower than in the US, but we are catching up. More than 100,000 Australian children are taking antidepressants[35] (mostly off label) and even more are on ADHD drugs, primarily amphetamines. This is despite the fact that the long-term evidence supporting these aggressive chemical interventions in developing brains and bodies is worse than weak.

Viewed from the perspective of patient and child wellbeing, this makes absolutely no sense. But if you accept the fundamental principle of economics – that self-interest drives most human and corporate behaviour – then it makes perfect sense. The APA, Big Pharma, and their collaborators in the USA, Australia and around the globe are acting in a totally rational way. Defining more people as mad and exaggerating the benefits and understating the risks of drugs, expands markets and grows profits. What could be more sane?

Each successive version of the DSM has involved 'diagnostic creep' – the loosening of diagnostic criteria for existing disorders or addition of new disorders. One notable exception to this pattern of diagnostic creep was the removal of the classification of homosexuality as a mental illness in the early 1970s. In 1952, the original DSM classified homosexuality as a 'sexual deviation disorder', as did the second edition, DSM-II, published in 1968. In December 1973, DSM-II was modified by the Board of Trustees of the APA. The Board voted to eliminate the general category of homosexuality and replace it with 'sexual orientation disturbance'. After this change, only individuals who were in conflict with their sexual orientation had a psychiatric disorder.[36]

This hard-fought victory over medicalised bigotry resulted from changing social norms and coordinated protest and lobbying. It is clear evidence that the development of the DSM has been driven by social, cultural and political considerations, rather than scientific advancement.

DSM-5's publication in May 2013 was a huge and controversial event within the psychiatric profession. There was significant international dissent in the lead up to its publication. Professor Allen Frances, the Chairman of the Task Force that developed the previous version, DSM-IV (published in 1994), led the backlash. With the benefit of hindsight, Frances regretted aspects of his own work on DSM-IV as having helped to trigger *'false epidemics' for autism and 'the wild over-diagnosis of attention deficit disorder'.*[37] *He wanted his successors to learn these lessons about the dangers of diagnostic creep and over-treatment.*

Instead, early drafts of DSM-5 included many reckless proposals that went beyond just proposing diagnostic creep and offered a diagnostic explosion that would have seen many millions of previously 'normal' people made potential psychiatric patients. As detailed in Chapter 3, Professor Frances argued passionately against the inclusion of 'pet disorders' pushed by enthusiastic researchers. The backlash he led caused the American Psychiatric Association to abandon, or tone down, some of its more controversial DSM-5 proposals, although many still made it into the published version.

Contests like this within the American psychiatric profession to dominate psychiatric practice has been likened to a 'two-party political system', with the Biological Party dominating the Environmental Party.[38] Biological Psychiatry attributes mental illness primarily to genetic predisposition and related undetectable biochemical brain imbalances. Environmental psychiatry (more commonly known as social psychiatry) emphasises non-biological individual circumstances like social isolation and trauma. Biological Psychiatry promotes diagnostic specificity and biochemical (pharmaceuticals and psychosurgery) treatments. Environmental Psychiatry places less emphasis on discrete diagnostic categories and promotes a range of behavioural interventions e.g. psychotherapy, peer counselling and cognitive behaviour therapy (CBT).

Seeking to understand the impact of anatomy, physiology, biochemistry and genetics on human behaviour is important scientific work that has the potential to benefit humankind. Biological Psychiatry is a legitimate field for scientific exploration but it is entirely illegitimate to pretend – as so many proponents of Biological Psychiatry do – that there is solid science when there is none.

Biological Psychiatry's increasing dominance has occurred during a period of massive scientific and technological breakthroughs. It is over fifty years since humankind's most celebrated technological achievement – sending men to the moon – created boundless optimism in the capacity of science to overcome all challenges. However, the challenge for Biological Psychiatry – understanding the interplay between brain, body and behaviour – is not rocket science; it is far more difficult.

It is also far more difficult than other aspects of modern medicine. Compared with what we know about the nature of physical disease, the science of Biological Psychiatry is best described as primitive. We simply do not know very much about how the human brain - the most complex object in the known universe with its estimated 86 billion neurons - works.[39] [40] The problem is that the pseudo-scientists who claim insights into the biological underpinnings of psychiatry massively overstate current scientific understandings of how our brain, bodies and behaviour interact. They act as if it they have access to the equivalent of a detailed street map of the brain when their understanding is more like an 18th Century atlas.

We know even less about the detail of how mental health drugs affect the brain and body particularly in the long-term. That has not stopped proponents of pseudo-scientific Biological Psychiatry arguing psychotropic (mind and behaviour altering) drugs like amphetamine for ADHD, and selective serotonin reuptake inhibitors (SSRIs) for depression, are the equivalent of Insulin for Diabetes.[41] Unlike diabetes, there are no blood tests, brain scans, genetic or other objective tests to confirm chemical imbalance hypotheses for any psychiatric disorder. All are diagnosed using behavioural criteria.

Despite the absence of diagnostic biomarkers, the central tenet of Biological Psychiatry is that psychiatric disorders are the result of genetic or other biological factors causing chemical imbalances in the brain. Physical health problems, trauma, social isolation, poverty, unemployment, lack of education, housing problems and alcohol and other drug problems are all drivers of poor mental health. But addressing these complex human needs is a lot more challenging than simply assuming that these problems result from, rather than cause, psychiatric disorders. It is far easier to simply apply a DSM diagnostic label and prescribe a pill, than to deal with an individual's unique circumstances.

The DSM is often referred to as the 'Bible of Psychiatry'. Rather than implying religious significance, the 'Bible' analogy is meant to reflect the DSM's dominant role in defining mental illness in many Western nations. However, much of modern psychiatric practice, particularly pharmaceutical psychiatry, is based on the belief (faith) that the underlying cause of mental illness is undetectable chemical imbalances in the brain. This 'faith-based' approach – which often ignores compelling contradictory evidence – suggests that the DSM Bible of Psychiatry analogy may be appropriate on two levels. In the absence of objective evidence, assuming that biological factors create chemical imbalances that cause aberrant behaviours (i.e. psychiatric disorders) is a leap of faith more characteristic of religion than science. [42] [43]

It is a leap of faith that the Royal Australia and New Zealand College of Psychiatry (RANZCP) promotes and the Australian Government endorses. The RANZCP website states that medications treat mental illness by rebalancing the chemicals in the brain.[44] The Australian Government goes even further. In 2007 it produced a series of brochures on anxiety, bipolar, depression, eating disorders, personality disorders and schizophrenia that are still available on the Australian Government Department of Health website.[45] All of these brochures declare that these conditions are believed to be caused by a chemical imbalance.

For example, the brochure *What is a depressive disorder?* states:

Depressive disorders are thought to be due, in part, to a chemical imbalance in the brain. Anti-depressant medication treats this imbalance... anti-depressant medications are not addictive. They slowly return the balance of neurotransmitters in the brain, taking one to four weeks to achieve their positive effects.[46]

The Government's claim that antidepressants are not addictive is grossly misleading. Many people who take antidepressants later regret it when they find they are very difficult – sometimes impossible – to withdraw from.[47] [48] After a prolonged argument, the UK Royal College of Psychiatry recently reluctantly conceded that what many patients were claiming is true, i.e. withdrawing from antidepressants is often a strange, frightening and torturous experience.[49] In contrast, the Australian Government continues to assert that antidepressants are not addictive and declare its faith in the ability of medications, to rebalance brain chemistry. Any drug company that claimed that antidepressants 'slowly return the balance of neurotransmitters in the brain' would be guilty of misleading promotion, but our Government continues to promote this lie.

Atheists and agnostics (like me) reject religion because we find the faith-based tenets of religions – virgin births, dead rising, reincarnation, alien spirits etc. – implausible. In contrast, the fundamental tenet of Biological Psychiatry – i.e. that biochemical brain imbalances cause mental illness – seems far more credible. It can be particularly appealing to those who strongly believe in the potential of science to think that human behaviour will be understood by reducing it to a series of soon-to-be understood chemical reactions. However, despite frequent over-hyped claims of imminent breakthroughs, we are nowhere near that level of understanding; and there is no guarantee we ever will be. Ironically the faith in reductionism inherent in Biological Psychiatry appears to be very attractive to some devout atheists.

Esoteric considerations aside, there is a very weak evidence base for many of the most common treatments used to treat DSM defined psychiatric disorders. It should not be good enough for mental health clinicians to speculate about possible specific biological causes and then base invasive treatment decisions on the assumption that they are correct. Medicine, and therefore psychiatry, must be held to a much higher standard of evidence. Faith in the existence of undetectable factors may be appropriate for religion, but not science and medicine.

Nonetheless, as it is currently practised Biological Psychiatry is a faith-based movement with a licence to chemically interfere with children. Can you imagine the outrage if other faith-based movements sought permission to drug children on the basis of hypothesised deficiencies? That is exactly what happens when we give children amphetamines to stop them fidgeting, playing too loudly, interrupting, and displaying the other ADHD diagnostic criteria. The rationale for this child abuse is the increasingly discredited hypothesis that ADHD is caused by malfunctioning dopamine receptors in the brain and that the 'therapeutic effect of stimulants is achieved by slow and steady increases of dopamine'.[50]

Paradoxically, there is evidence that long term exposure to the amphetamines and amphetamine-type stimulants to treat ADHD may cause dopamine system malfunctions that never existed before.[51] In other words, the drugs used to treat ADHD can create the condition that is hypothesised as causing ADHD. In the case of ADHD, the use of amphetamines to treat hypothetical chemical imbalances, to manage behaviour, is more like a cult than a religion.[52] Yet this cult-like behaviour is officially endorsed and sponsored by governments, not just in Australia but also in most developed countries around the globe.

The evolution of the DSM reflects the long-term commercial realities of American psychiatry. Psychologists, counsellors and social workers are all able to offer professional talking therapies as alternatives to psychiatry. Even friends and family can offer informal chats and advice. The licence to medically intervene either pharmacologically or through surgery is psychiatry's major marketing edge. It makes perfect sense for the APA to be in bed with Big Pharma. Both benefit from promoting medical interventions (primarily drugs) rather than less invasive talking therapies.

According to a prominent critic of the pharmaceuticalisation of mental health, American psychiatrist Peter Breggin:

> In the 1970s, the APA was going broke. Many psychiatrists were having difficulty filling their practices. Always near the bottom of the medical income scale, psychiatrists were floundering economically. Competition from non-medical professionals was cutting heavily into private practices…In the early 1980s, the APA made a decision that changed its history and that of our society. It decided to create an economic and political partnership with the drug companies. The partnership would enable psychiatry to use drug company funds to promote the medical model, psychopharmacology, and the authority and

influence of psychiatry. Backed by the multi-billion dollar drug industry, psychiatry hoped to defeat the threat from non-medical professionals, such as psychologists and social workers. Within a scant few years, APA transformed itself from a failing institution into one of the most powerful political forces in the nation. It developed lobbying groups in state capitals and in Washington, DC; gained a stronger influence in the media and the courts; and distributed increasing numbers of drugs to escalating numbers of people. Psychiatry's decision to save itself by going into partnership with the drug companies was an openly discussed survival plan.[53]

Even within the American Psychiatric Association, questions have long been asked about the appropriateness of their relationship with the pharmaceutical industry. In 1985 Dr Fred Gottlieb, APA Speaker of the House, told the APA:

I do not suggest that either they [the drug companies] or we [the American Psychiatric Association] are evil folks. But I continue to believe that accepting such money is, in the long run, inimical to our independent functioning. We have evolved a somewhat casual and quite cordial relationship with the drug houses, taking their money readily...We seem to discount available data that drug advertising promotes irrational prescribing practices. We seem to think that we as psychiatrists are immune from the kinds of unconscious emotional bias in favour of those who are overtly friendly toward us...We persist in ignoring an inherent conflict of interest.[54]

This unhealthily close relationship has led Big Pharma and American Psychiatry to treat depression, schizophrenia, ADHD and many other psychiatric disorders as if they are caused by a biochemical imbalance.

In 2000, Harvard University Medical School psychiatrist and author Joseph Glenmullen stated: 'In every instance where such an imbalance was thought to have been found, it was later proven false'.[55] Worse still, the psychiatric drugs, particularly antipsychotics, used to treat hypothesised biochemical imbalances frequently create biochemical imbalances and brain damage.[56]

None of this appears to matter to the APA. Dr Harold Pincus, Vice Chairman of the DSM-IV Development Task Force, was quoted in 2000 as saying, 'There has never been any criterion that psychiatric diagnoses require a demonstrated biological aetiology [cause]'.[57] Twenty years later and this has not changed. There has been a gentle adjustment in the language used by some proponents of Pseudo-Scientific Biological Psychiatry. Some still use the term chemical imbalance[58], however, it is now more common to suggest that genetic neuro-developmental factors underpin mental illness.

These assertions about the biological causes of mental illness remain speculation and the dominant treatment of psychiatric disorders is still chemicals used in the hope that they adjust brain chemistry in an appropriate manner. Clearly the APA thinks that it is not crucial to understand the causes of psychiatric problems. However, causes do matter. Regardless of whether the discipline is medicine, economics, politics or any field of human endeavour, to solve a problem, it is best to understand its cause.

It is the failure to care about causes that has resulted in psychiatry, more than every other medical discipline, being spectacularly unsuccessful at finding cures. In fact the only psychiatric disorder eradicated by the APA was 'sexual deviation disorder'. This was of course because political and public pressure forced the APA to eventually concede that there was nothing to cure and reluctantly acknowledge that homosexuality is difference not disease.

The APA clearly learned very little from this experience. Instead it has accelerated its pattern of turning difference into disease. Playing loudly, fidgeting, disliking homework, climbing and running excessively, 'being on the go as if driven by a motor' are no longer just childhood behaviours. The APA has made them the diagnostic criteria of a neuro-developmental psychiatric disorder i.e. ADHD. In the case of ADHD, out of nothing the APA has created a massive industry with global market sales for 'ADHD medications' valued at an estimated US$16.4 billion in 2018, and forecast to be worth US$24.9 billion by 2025.[59] These figures do not include the payments received for diagnosing, researching, promoting and providing non-drug treatments, so the ADHD industry is considerably larger. Nonetheless, the 2018 value of drug sales alone was larger than the national income (GDP) of 68 of the 186 countries for which the International Monetary Fund provided 2018 data. In fact, it was bigger than the combined GDP of 19 of the world's smallest economies.[60]

Evidence of Big Pharma's corrupting influence on the APA was revealed in 2008, when the US Senate Finance Committee, driven by Republican Senator Charles Grassley, began an investigation into the APA financial ties to the pharmaceutical industry. Senator Grassley's probing revealed that in 2006 the pharmaceutical industry accounted for about 30% of the APA's US$62.5 million annual revenue. About half of that money went to drug advertisements in psychiatric journals and exhibits at the annual meeting, and the other half to sponsor fellowships, conferences and industry symposiums at the annual meeting. It was also revealed that more than half the psychiatrists that developed the DSM-IV had previously received drug company funding. This pattern was repeated for DSM-5. Three quarters of the DSM-5 working groups had a majority of 'members with financial ties to the pharmaceutical industry'. As with the DSM-IV, the 'most conflicted panels' were those for which drug treatments are the 'first-line intervention'.[61]

In light of Senator Grassley's revelations, the corrupting influence of Big Pharma money was recognised at the top level of the APA in July 2008 by President Dr Steven S. Sharfstein:

> With every new revelation, our credibility with patients has been damaged, and we have to protect that first and foremost...I think we need to review all arrangements between doctors and industry and be very clear about what constitutes a conflict of interest and what does not.[62]

A month later, and shortly before he retired as APA President, Dr Sharfstein wrote a ground-breaking commentary piece on the relationship between psychiatry and the pharmaceutical industry titled *Big Pharma and American Psychiatry: the Good, the Bad, and the Ugly*:

> Financial incentives and managed care have contributed to the notion of a 'quick fix' by taking a pill and reducing the emphasis on psychotherapy and psychosocial treatments... We must work hard to end this situation and get involved in advocacy to reform our health care system from the bottom up. There are examples of the 'ugly' practices that undermine the credibility of our profession. Drug company representatives will be the first to say that it is the doctors who request the fancy dinners, cruises, tickets to athletic events, and so on. But can we really be surprised that several states have passed laws to force disclosure of these gifts? So-called 'preceptorships' are another example of the 'ugly'; that is, drug companies who pay physicians to allow company reps to sit in on patient sessions allegedly to learn more about care for patients and then advise the doctor on appropriate prescribing. Drug company representatives bearing gifts are frequent visitors to psychiatrists' offices and consulting rooms. We should have the wisdom and distance to call these gifts what they are – kickbacks and bribes.[63]

Sharfstein's 2008 comments were similar to the comments by APA Speaker of the House Fred Gottlieb some twenty-three years prior, however, his honest appraisal temporarily gave hope of a fresh approach, where patient needs were the primary focus of psychiatric practice. The development of DSM-5, which was eventually published in 2013, dashed these hopes.

Chapter 3

From Bad to Worse, DSM-5 replaces DSM-IV

The DSM is now 68 years old, and the pattern of diagnostic creep began well before DSM-5. This is freely admitted by Professor Allen Frances, the psychiatrist who led the development of DSM-IV – the prior edition – that was published in 1994. Taking responsibility for past mistakes can be especially problematic for members of the American medical profession, who work within a blame avoidance culture created by the ever-present threat of malpractice suits. Special praise is therefore due to Professor Frances for his efforts to ensure that the mistakes of DSM-IV were acknowledged and not repeated in the development of DSM-5.[64] Of course, Professor Frances was not solely responsible for the development of DSM-IV, and it is likely DSM-IV would have been significantly worse if not for his leadership. However, as the overall leader of the DSM-IV development process, he has accepted his share of responsibility for the problems DSM-IV helped create.

In a very public about-turn, Professor Frances became the unofficial leader of an international fight against the disease-mongering (new disorders and looser diagnostic criteria for existing disorders) central to the development of DSM-5. There were some successes in this fight. Most notably, the APA eventually retreated from plans to include Psychosis Risk Disorder (see Chapter 5) and abandoned some of its more extreme planned changes to the diagnostic criteria for ADHD (see Chapter 6). However, the APA pushed on with most of its proposed changes.

When the final version of DSM-5 was formally endorsed by the Board of Trustees of the APA, Professor Frances wrote the following opinion piece that eloquently expresses the concerns of many critics of the DSM-5.

DSM-5 Is a Guide, Not a Bible: Simply Ignore Its 10 Worst Changes

Edited version of a Huff Post blog written by Professor Allen Frances, 12 March 2012[65].

> This is the saddest moment in my 45 year career of studying, practicing, and teaching psychiatry... My best advice to clinicians, to the press, and to the general public – be skeptical and don't follow DSM-5 blindly down a road likely to lead to massive over-diagnosis and harmful over-medication. Just ignore the ten changes that make no sense...DSM-5 got off to a bad start and was never able to establish sure footing. Its leaders initially articulated a premature and unrealizable goal- to produce a paradigm shift in psychiatry. Excessive ambition combined with disorganized execution led inevitably to many ill-conceived and risky proposals. These were vigorously opposed. More than fifty mental health professional associations petitioned for an outside review of DSM-5 to provide an independent judgment of its supporting evidence and to evaluate the balance between its risks and benefits. Professional journals, the press, and the public also weighed in – expressing widespread astonishment about decisions that sometimes seemed not only to lack scientific support but also to defy common sense.
>
> DSM-5 has neither been able to self-correct nor willing to heed the

advice of outsiders. It has instead created a mostly closed shop – circling the wagons and deaf to the repeated and widespread warnings that it would lead to massive misdiagnosis. Fortunately, some of its most egregiously risky and unsupportable proposals were eventually dropped under great external pressure... But [the] APA stubbornly refused to sponsor any independent review and has given final approval to the ten reckless and untested ideas that are summarized below.

The history of psychiatry is littered with fad diagnoses that in retrospect did far more harm than good. Yesterday's APA approval makes it likely that DSM-5 will start a half or dozen or more new fads which will be detrimental to the misdiagnosed individuals and costly to our society...

There is an inherent and influential conflict of interest between the DSM-5 public trust and DSM-5 as a best seller. When its deadlines were consistently missed due to poor planning and disorganized implementation, APA chose quietly to cancel the DSM-5 field testing step that was meant to provide it with a badly needed opportunity for quality control. The current draft has been approved and is now being rushed prematurely to press with incomplete field testing for one reason only – so that DSM-5 publishing profits can fill the big hole in APA's projected budget and return dividends on the exorbitant cost of 25 million dollars that has been charged to DSM-5 preparation.

This is no way to prepare or to approve a diagnostic system. Psychiatric diagnosis has become too important in selecting treatments, determining eligibility for benefits and services, allocating resources, guiding legal judgments, creating stigma, and influencing personal expectations to be left in the hands of an APA that has proven itself incapable of producing a safe, sound, and widely accepted manual.

New diagnoses in psychiatry are more dangerous than new drugs because they influence whether or not millions of people are placed on drugs – often by primary care doctors after brief visits. Before their introduction, new diagnoses deserve the same level of attention to safety that we devote to new drugs. APA is not competent to do this.

So, here is my list of DSM-5's ten most potentially harmful changes. I would suggest that clinicians not follow these at all (or, at the very least, use them with extreme caution and attention to their risks); that potential patients be deeply skeptical, especially if the proposed diagnosis is being used as a rationale for prescribing medication for you or for your child; and that payers question whether some of these are suitable for reimbursement. My goal is to minimize the harm that may otherwise be done by unnecessary obedience to unwise and arbitrary DSM-5 decisions.

1. **Disruptive Mood Dysregulation Disorder**: DSM-5 will turn temper tantrums into a mental disorder – a puzzling decision based on the work of only one research group. We have no idea whatever how this untested new diagnosis will play out in real life practice settings, but my fear is that it will exacerbate, not relieve, the already excessive and inappropriate use of medication in young children. During the past two decades, child psychiatry has already provoked three fads – a tripling of Attention Deficit Disorder, a more than twenty-times increase in Autistic Disorder, and a forty-times increase in childhood Bipolar Disorder. The field should have felt chastened by this sorry track record and should engage itself now in the crucial task of educating practitioners and the public about the difficulty of accurately diagnosing children and the risks of over-medicating them. DSM-5 should not be adding a new disorder likely to result in a new fad and even more inappropriate medication use in vulnerable children.

2. **Normal** grief **will become Major Depressive Disorder**, thus medicalizing and trivializing our expectable and necessary emotional reactions to the loss of a loved one and substituting pills and superficial medical rituals for the deep consolations of family, friends, religion, and the resiliency that comes with time and the acceptance of the limitations of life.

3. The everyday forgetting characteristic of old age will now be misdiagnosed as **Minor Neurocognitive Disorder**, creating a huge false positive population of people who are not at special risk for dementia. Since there is no effective treatment for this 'condition' (or for dementia), the label provides absolutely no benefit (while creating great anxiety) even for those at true risk for later developing dementia. It is a dead loss for the many who will be mislabeled.

4. DSM-5 will likely trigger a fad of **Adult Attention Deficit Disorder** leading to widespread misuse of stimulant drugs for performance enhancement and recreation and contributing to the already large illegal secondary market in diverted prescription drugs.

5. Excessive eating 12 times in 3 months is no longer just a manifestation of gluttony and the easy availability of really great tasting food. DSM-5 has instead turned it into a psychiatric illness called Binge Eating **Disorder**.

6. The changes in the DSM-5 definition of Autism will result in lowered rates – 10% according to estimates by the DSM-5 work group, perhaps 50% according to outside research groups. This reduction can be seen as beneficial in the sense that the diagnosis of Autism will be more accurate and specific – but advocates understandably fear a disruption in

needed school services. Here the DSM 5 problem is not so much a bad decision, but the misleading promises that it will have no impact on rates of disorder or of service delivery. School services should be tied more to educational need, less to a controversial psychiatric diagnosis created or clinical (not educational) purposes and whose rate is so sensitive to small changes in definition and assessment.

7. **First time substance abusers will be lumped in definitionally in with hard core addicts** despite their very different treatment needs and prognosis and the stigma this will cause.

8. DSM-5 has created a slippery slope by introducing the concept of **Behavioral Addictions** that eventually can spread to make a mental disorder of everything we like to do a lot. Watch out for careless overdiagnosis of internet and sex addiction and the development of lucrative treatment programs to exploit these new markets.

9. DSM-5 obscures the already fuzzy boundary between Generalized Anxiety Disorder and the worries of everyday life. Small changes in definition can create millions of anxious new 'patients' and expand the already widespread practice of inappropriately prescribing addicting anti-anxiety medications.

10. DSM-5 has opened the gate even further to the already existing problem of misdiagnosis of PTSD in forensic settings.

DSM 5 has dropped its pretension to being a paradigm shift in psychiatric diagnosis and instead (in a dramatic 180 degree turn) now makes the equally misleading claim that it is a conservative document that will have minimal impact on the rates of psychiatric diagnosis and in the consequent provision of inappropriate treatment. This is an untenable claim that DSM 5 cannot possibly support because, for completely unfathomable reasons, it never took the simple and inexpensive step of actually studying the impact of DSM on rates in real world settings.

Except for autism, all the DSM 5 changes loosen diagnosis and threaten to turn our current diagnostic inflation into diagnostic hyperinflation. Painful experience with previous DSM's teaches that if anything in the diagnostic system can be misused and turned into a fad, it will be. Many millions of people with normal grief, gluttony, distractibility, worries, reactions to stress, the temper tantrums of childhood, the forgetting of old age, and 'behavioral addictions' will soon be mislabeled as psychiatrically sick and given inappropriate treatment.

People with real psychiatric problems that can be reliably diagnosed and effectively treated are already badly short-changed. DSM 5 will make this worse by diverting attention and scarce resources away from the really ill and toward people with the everyday problems of life who will be harmed, not helped, when they are mislabelled as mentally ill.

Our patients deserve better, society deserves better, and the mental health professions deserve better. Caring for the mentally ill is a noble and effective profession. But we have to know our limits and stay within them. DSM 5 violates the most sacred (and most frequently ignored) tenet in medicine- First Do No Harm! That is why this is such a sad moment.[66]

From an Australian perspective, the most disappointing aspect of DSM-5 was the limp reaction of health authorities, our political leaders, and the relevant professional bodies including the Australian

Medical Association (AMA), the Royal Australian College of General Practitioners (RACGP), and especially the Royal Australian and New Zealand College of Psychiatry (RANZCP).

The RANZCP as the organisation representing specialists in psychiatry failed its obligation to patients to properly scrutinise DSM-5. By keeping their critical analysis of the DSM-5 to a bare minimum[67] and then embracing DSM-5 as the definitive diagnostic guide for psychiatric disorders[68], the RANZCP has smoothed the transition from DSM-IV to DSM-5 and endorsed the APA's psychiatric disease-mongering. As a consequence, hundreds of thousands, possibly millions, of ordinary Australian who under DSM-IV were 'sane' now meet the criteria for at least one of the APA's 312 disorders. It is hard to think of a more significant case of cultural surrender. In effect, the Australian psychiatric profession let a group of American shrinks, awash with Big Pharma money, define what is acceptable, what is normal; and what is unacceptable, what is insane.

There was some critical analysis in the Australian media prior to DSM-5's publication, driven by psychiatrists Jon Jureidini, David Castle, Tim Carey and psychiatric epidemiologist Melissa Raven. To the best of my knowledge, I – at the time a WA State Parliamentary opposition backbencher – was the only politician to express concern about DSM-5. Apart from generating media that possibly contributed to the global backlash that moderated a few of the extreme proposals in early drafts of the DSM-5, it is hard to make the case that our collective activism had any local impact. Whether it was apathy – a modern version of 'no worries, she'll be right' – or the influence of vested interests working behind the scenes to smooth the transition, is not clear. But what is certain is that DSM-5 replaced DSM-IV with a minimum of fuss and next to no scrutiny, and overnight millions of previously officially 'sane' people in Australia and around the globe had undiagnosed psychiatric disorders.

Take the DSM-5 Challenge – how many psychiatric disorders do you have?

Borrow a copy of the DSM-5 (don't buy one – the American Psychiatric Association don't deserve your money) and browse it for 30 minutes to see how many psychiatric disorders you have qualified for. Over the course of my lifetime, I would have at various ages qualified for a diagnosis of persistent ADHD, Oppositional Defiant Disorder, Social Anxiety Disorder, Binge Eating Disorder, Alcohol Use Disorder and intermittent Insomnia Disorder. If you can't find at least three disorders that you would have qualified for, then I would suggest you are not normal, and possibly qualify for DDD (Disorder Deficit Disorder). In addition, if having browsed the DSM-5, you consider these diagnoses 'scientific', you likely have comorbid CSDD (Common Sense Deficit Disorder).

There is a ready-made alternative to the APA's DSM. Although the DSM is becoming increasingly influential around the globe, the World Health Organization's *International Clarification of Diseases* 10 (ICD-10) has provided the diagnostic criteria for mental health disorders predominantly used in Europe. Despite the fact that Australia is a member of the World Health Organization and obviously not a member of the American Psychiatric Association, DSM criteria are the predominant criteria used in Australia.

Unlike the DSM – which deals only with mental illness – ICD covers the complete range of medical conditions and physical illness. Chapter 5 of the ICD details the diagnostic criteria of psychiatric disorders and provides a numerical code that can be used to identify a disorder when clinicians claim payment from health insurers and government authorities. The ICD-10 numerical coding system is often used in the Australian health system by clinicians and hospitals to obtain Medicare co-payment entitlements; however, DSM-5 is the most commonly used diagnostic system.[69]

The development of the ICD has tended to lag the DSM in reflecting the shift within psychiatry from a psychoanalytic approach (emphasising personal historical circumstances and later consequences) to a system that defines behavioural symptoms of an increasing number of discreet, although often comorbid (co-existing), disorders. Despite a gradual convergence, significant but subtle differences remain. While many of the criticisms of the subjectivity of assessment of behaviours are common to both systems, the DSM generally contains looser, less rigorous diagnostic criteria than the ICD. A 2005 study compared diagnosis rates for a range of childhood psychiatric disorders using the diagnostic criteria in DSM-IV and the equivalent disorder in ICD-10. For the majority of disorders, rates of diagnosis were higher using DSM-IV.[70]

DSM-5's publication in 2013 further widened the gap between the two systems. ICD-11 is due for publication in 2022. Perhaps the gap will close up a little again then; however, the DSM has always promoted more extreme disease mongering than the ICD. Although it is far from perfect, if we as a nation chose to use the WHO's ICD rather than the APA's DSM, this would instantaneously mean hundreds of thousands of Aussies are no longer officially mentally ill. A shift from the DSM to the ICD would likely be very good for patients, but it would not be good for drug company sales.

Not surprisingly since the publication of DSM-5, Australian rates of psychotropic medication use have grown rapidly.

Growth in Australian psychotropic prescribing rates since DSM-5 was published in 2013

Antidepressants: the number of Australians on antidepressants was already high. In the period July 2012 to June 2013, 2,490,793 Australians (about 10.9%) were prescribed an antidepressant. For the period July 2017 to June 2018, this figure rose to 3,042,922

(12.2%). The fastest growth was for children (aged 0-17) with the number rising from 69,973 (1.3%) to 101,174 (1.8%).[71]

Antipsychotics: According to SANE Australia, 'in 2011, nearly 350,000 Australians had at least one prescription filled for antipsychotic medication. That's 1.6% of the population'.[72]

In the period July 2017 until June 2018, the number of Australians prescribed at least one script had risen to 406,999 (roughly 1.7%).[73] The vast majority (73%) of this prescribing was done by GPs.

The fastest growth appears to be for children. According to News Corp, 'Federal health department data… show[s] the number of children aged 17 or under prescribed antipsychotics increased by 24 per cent between 2013-14 [from 19,934] and 2017-18 [to 24,700], far outstripping the age group's 5 per cent population growth'.[74]

ADHD medications (primarily amphetamines): In 2013, 75,386 Australian children (approximately 1.9% of those aged 4 to 17) were prescribed an ADHD drug. By 2017, this number grew to 107,345. Since 2017 rates of prescribing have grown about 11% per annum. In 2019, it is estimated that approximately 130,000 children (3.0% of those aged 4-17) were prescribed an ADHD drug. From 2013 to 2019, the number of Australian adults prescribed an ADHD drug grew from 37,159 to approximately 70,000.

These high and rapidly growing rates of prescription psychotropic drug use are an inevitable consequence of outsourcing our definitions of insanity to the USA and embracing a culture that values superficiality and quick fixes. Australia's almost unconscious adoption of DSM-5 is cultural capture at its most extreme.

Usually Australian psychiatric practise lags the USA by five to 10 years; however, as detailed in Chapter 4, in relation to antidepressant use, Australia is ahead of the pack (but not in a good way).

Chapter 4

Antidepressants, Youth Suicide and Self-Harm – the Depressing Truth

The most troubling aspect of Australian psychiatric practice is how little attention is paid to the obligation to 'first do no harm'. Too often, practitioners assume the best about their interventions – drug treatments and psychosurgery – and the worst about their patients. If a patient has terrible outcomes after treatment, typically this is assumed to be an inevitable part of the course of mental illness and that outcomes would be even worse without treatment. The possibility of iatrogenic harm is summarily dismissed. The most disturbing local example of this is the pattern of wilful ignorance displayed in relation to the use of antidepressants and the incidence of suicide and self-harm by young Australians.

In Australia, no antidepressant is approved for the treatment of depression or anxiety in people aged under 18 years, and there is increasing evidence that antidepressants have very little benefit in treating depression in young people.[75] [76] Nonetheless, from July 2017 to June 2018, 101,174 (approximately 1.8%) of Australians aged 0-17 were prescribed an antidepressant.

Two selective serotonin reuptake inhibitors (SSRI) antidepressants, fluvoxamine and sertraline (brand name Zoloft), are approved in Australia for children and adolescents with obsessive compulsive disorder.[77] However, the first *Australian Atlas of Healthcare Variation*, published in 2015, suggested that, for most children, antidepressants are 'primarily prescribed for anxiety' and secondarily for depression.[78] The vast majority of SSRI and other antidepressant prescribing for children in Australia is therefore 'off label'. As a 2019 *Lancet* editorial on off label prescribing concluded:

> Children are not small adults and evidence-based treatment is arguably even more important in children. Both the potential for adverse events with lifelong consequences and the danger of ineffective drugs with poor outcomes have far-reaching consequences.[79]

FDA + TGA Suicidality Warnings

In October 2004, the US Food and Drug Administration (FDA) issued a black box warning (the highest level of warning) that using antidepressants was associated with an increased risk of suicidal thinking and behaviour in people under 18 years of age with depression and other psychiatric disorders. In 2007, the warning was expanded to include young adults under 25 years of age.[80] [81] The warning was a result of an FDA analysis of short-term trials of antidepressants in children and adolescents that showed 'a relative risk for suicidal behaviour or ideation of 1.95 (95% confidence interval 1.28 to 2.98) for those treated with antidepressants compared with those given placebo'.[82] However, as discussed below, the FDA warning was strongly criticised by some prominent US psychiatrists.[83]

In August 2005, in response to the FDA's 2004 black box warning, the Australian Government's medical product safety regulator, the Therapeutic Goods Administration (TGA), stopped short of issuing the equivalent Boxed Warning. Instead the TGA required the rewording of Product Information and Consumer Information leaflets, which are made available to doctors and consumers respectively, to inform them of the need to monitor for signs of suicidality.[84] This light regulatory approach was typical of the TGA at that time. From January to September 2005, the FDA issued twenty black box warnings for prescription drugs that were sold in both the US and Australia, but the TGA issued equivalent warnings for only five of them.[85] As detailed in Chapter 8, the TGA's soft touch regulatory approach continues today.

Our local 'experts' challenge the FDA warning

Subsequent to the FDA's black box warning and the TGA's lower-level warnings, several prominent Australian mental health advocacy organisations and influential Australian psychiatrists disputed the antidepressant-youth suicidality nexus, and claimed that the use of antidepressants, on balance, reduced the risk of youth suicide. The most disturbing example is *Suicide Prevention Australia*, our self-declared *'national peak body for the suicide prevention sector'*.[86] It has received substantial and increasing funding from successive Australian Governments to provide guidance on, and conduct research into suicide prevention.

In 2010, *Suicide Prevention Australia* published a *Youth Suicide Prevention* position statement, which concluded that, 'balanced against the risk of not treating youth depression, SSRIs [the most common form of antidepressants prescribed in Australia] offer some potential to reduce youth suicide'.[87] *Suicide Prevention Australia's* position statement cited only a single source, Gould et al.'s (2003) literature review spanning 1992 to 2002, to support its positive risk assessment, claiming that it had 'shown [SSRIs] to be an effective treatment for youth depression and suicidality'. In fact, Gould et al. had only said it was 'plausible' that increased antidepressant prescribing might have decreased youth suicide rates.[88]

Suicide Prevention Australia's position statement also stated that 'the decreased use of SSRIs in Australia has recently been linked to increased youth suicides', but identified no evidence of an Australian decrease in use of SSRIs and no basis for the alleged link with youth suicide.[89] In fact, as detailed later in this chapter, in the period between the FDA warning and *Suicide Prevention Australia* producing its position statement, among young Australians a substantial fall in antidepressant prescribing rates was associated with a small fall in the suicide rate.

The next sentence in the *Suicide Prevention Australia* position statement cited a highly credible Cochrane review[90] of SSRI antidepressant use by children and adolescents as supporting fluoxetine (common brand Prozac) as the 'most effective SSRI'.[91] However, the Cochrane review reported that, even for fluoxetine, 'the reduction seen in symptoms was modest' and the limited evidence came from trials of 'young people not representative of those presenting for treatment in clinics'.[92] The *Suicide Prevention Australia* position statement did not report that the Cochrane review found 'an increased risk of suicidal ideation and behaviour' and higher rates of adverse events among children and adolescents prescribed SSRIs compared with placebo.[93]

In summary, Australia's peak body on suicide prevention made unreferenced claims, misrepresented or ignored the findings of research it cited, and minimised the importance of the FDA and TGA suicidality warnings. In March 2019, nearly a decade after its publication, *Suicide Prevention Australia* removed the position statement from its website.[94]

In 2010, when *Suicide Prevention Australia* published its position paper, 320 young Australians (aged under 25 years) suicided. Since then the number and per-capita rate of youth suicide has steadily increased. In 2019 the total number of deaths by suicide for Australians aged under

25 years was 480.[95] *Suicide Prevention Australia* has clearly failed young Australians, but this has not hurt it financially. In the 2019 financial year *Suicide Prevention Australia* had revenue of $4,882,879, and produced a surplus of $417,551, mostly derived from taxpayer funds. From 30 June 2012 (the earliest data available), until 30 June 2019, SPA's net worth increased from $178,535 to $2,321,893.[96] [97]

Suicide Prevention Australia's position statement also cited a 2009 *Evidence Summary: Using SSRI Antidepressants to Treat Depression in Young People: What are the Issues and What is the Evidence?* produced by influential Australian non-government mental health organisations, Orygen and headspace.[98] Orygen runs a clinical service in Melbourne and focusses heavily on research.[99] The establishment of both Orygen and headspace – which runs more than 130 mental health clinics across Australia targeting 12-25-year-olds – was driven by Professor Patrick McGorry. Both headspace and Orygen are funded primarily by government. McGorry was listed as a clinical adviser on the Evidence Summary.

The *Evidence Summary* noted that no antidepressant was approved for use by under-18 year-olds for the treatment of depression, and acknowledged the FDA warning, however, it concluded that there were 'even greater risks of not treating depression with any type of intervention (e.g. pharmacological or psychological)'.[100] This statement groups together drug and talking therapies with very different harm-benefit profiles, and provides no evidence for or against either type of treatment.

The 2009 Evidence Summary (and the updated 2015 version[101]) stated that, of all SSRI antidepressants, fluoxetine is superior, but even it is only 'modestly effective for reducing symptoms of depression in young people'.[102] Nonetheless, it recommended that SSRIs may be used to treat moderate to severe depression 'within the context of comprehensive management of the patient, which includes regular careful monitoring for the emergence of suicidal ideation or behaviour'. [103]

Orygen – do as we say, not as we did (or do?)

Despite these words of caution about the need for 'regular careful monitoring' an audit of the prescribing practices at Orygen's own clinic demonstrated that it had not practiced what it preached. In 2007 at Orygen 'the majority of young people (74.5%) were prescribed an antidepressant before an adequate trial of psychotherapy was undertaken and that less than 50% were monitored for depression symptom improvement and antidepressant treatment emergent suicide related behaviours (35% and 30% respectively)'.[104] Results of this audit were not published until 2012[105] and there is no publicly available evidence of subsequent prescribing audits, so we can have no confidence that Orygen has improved its practices since 2007.

Adding to these concerns about Orygen's prescribing practices is the fact that in February 2009, the same year that Orygen produced the original Evidence Summary, it also published a document *Medications for Depression* that made no reference to suicidality risks, and contradicted the Evidence Summary by overstating the evidence for the effectiveness of antidepressants. *Medications for Depression* states: 'Antidepressants also work well for less severe types of depression', whereas the Orygen/headspace Evidence Summary states that, of all SSRI antidepressants, only 'fluoxetine is modestly effective for reducing symptoms of depression in young people'.[106] Despite this inaccuracy, *Medications for Depression* was still available on Orygen's website (as at 6 April 2020).[107] It was only removed from Orygen's website after there was widespread media coverage[108] [109] of a journal article co-authored by me, Melissa Raven and Jon Jureidini that included criticism of *Medications for Depression*.[110]

Ian Hickie – Australia's depression guru

Professor Ian Hickie is arguably Australia's most influential Australian depression expert. In 2000, Hickie was appointed as the inaugural CEO of beyondblue: the national depression initiative, a prominent mental health organisation funded by the Commonwealth and state governments. He rapidly developed a high profile in the media, and he was appointed to numerous government and NGO committees, boards, and working groups. In 2006, he was named by the *Australian Financial Review* in its list of Australia's top 10 cultural influencers for his leadership in mental health and depression in particular.[111] (See Chapter 7 for more detail.)

In 2003, the year before the FDA issued its warning, Hickie was a co-author of a frequently quoted study (Hall et al. 2003), supporting the use of SSRI antidepressants. The abstract concluded:

> Changes in suicide rates and exposure to antidepressants in Australia for 1991-2000 are significantly associated. This effect is most apparent in older age groups, in which rates of suicide decreased substantially in association with exposure to antidepressants. The increase in antidepressant prescribing may be a proxy marker for improved overall management of depression. If so, increased prescribing of selective serotonin reuptake inhibitors in general practice may have produced a quantifiable benefit in population mental health.[112]

However, the results, detailed in the body of Hall and Hickie et al. 2003, are inconsistent with the abstract's positive conclusions. The results show that over the period of the study (1986 to 2000) there was a massive increase in antidepressant prescribing for all ages and an increase of approximately 16% in the per-capita suicide rate for Australians aged 15 to 45. While there was a 15% fall in the per-capita suicide rate for Australians aged 45 or older, when combined, the per-capita suicide rate for all Australians (aged 15 or older) rose by 3%. Because of the growth in suicides among Australians aged 15 to 44 (who made up 59% of the population of Australia aged 15 or older), the life-years lost to suicide will have risen by significantly more than 3%. How Hall and Hickie reached such positive conclusions and why a reputable journal like the BMJ allowed such a flawed abstract to be printed is a mystery.

Hickie compounded the problems with Hall et al (2003) when he cited it on several occasions, one as recent as 2019[113], as evidence that increasing antidepressant use rates are associated with better treatment outcomes and fewer suicides.[114] [115] For example, in a 2007 BMJ debate piece he cited it as evidence of an inverse causal effect, writing that 'increased treatment of depression reduces suicides'. Hickie also asserted:

> Although there has been much hype and regulatory concern about increased prescribing of the new drugs [SSRIs], there is little hard evidence of harm to a significant number of people. The real harm, as evidenced by the suicide statistics, comes from not receiving a diagnosis or treatment when you have a life threatening condition like depression.[116]

In a similar vein, in a May 2010 televised debate, *Is Depression Being Over-Diagnosed?*, Hickie ridiculed as 'absolute total nonsense' the assertion by psychiatrist Dr Tanveer Ahmed that, on occasion, normal sadness was being pathologised, and depression was being over-diagnosed and over-treated with medications. He went on to praise growing rates of medication use and psychological treatments. Hickie concluded, 'when depression's been treated, suicide goes down, in this country, and many other countries – well demonstrated!'[117] Despite the assertive and dismissive tone Professor Hickie used towards Dr Ahmed, it is clear it wasn't Dr Ahmed who was talking 'absolute total nonsense'.

Later in 2010, Professors McGorry and Hickie co-authored an opinion piece on youth depression in the *Medical Journal of Australia* that had significant errors which created the impression that antidepressant use was on balance likely to prevent youth suicide.[118]

Analysis of Professor Hickie and McGorry's opinion piece
Guidelines for youth depression: time to incorporate new perspectives. MJA (2010)

Hickie and McGorry's opinion piece cited *Gibbons et al. 2006*[119] as evidence that in the US, following the October 2004 FDA warning, a fall in antidepressant prescribing 'was associated with an increase in suicides in young people'.[120] That was nonsense. The figures in this study came from 1996-1998, years before any black box warning or decrease in prescribing.

Professors Hickie and McGorry may have intended to refer to another USl study by Gibbons et al., published in 2007.[121] However, that study incorrectly associated a 22% decrease in SSRI prescriptions with a 14% increase in US youth suicide rates between 2003 and 2004. In fact, in 2004, the year in which suicide rates rose, there was no significant drop in SSRI prescribing; this did not occur until 2005 when youth suicide rates actually fell.[122]

Hickie and McGorry also wrote: 'Previous population-based data have indicated a positive relationship between exposure to antidepressants and reduction in suicides'.[123] They cited Simon et al.[124] as evidence that 'most [under-18] suicide attempts occur in the month before treatment and then decline sharply once treatment has commenced'[125], without acknowledging that Simon et al. reported only on adolescents treated with antidepressants. As suicide attempts are a common trigger for initiating antidepressant treatment, this sharp decline would be expected. It is certainly not evidence that antidepressants reduce suicide risk.

These sorts of flawed papers by prominent psychiatric thought leaders like Professors Hickie and McGorry matter. They are not just of academic interest, they affect policy and practice, and therefore they affect lives.

For example, Hall et al. (2003) influenced the TGA's 2005 response to the FDAs initial 2004 black box warning. In its response, *Suicidality with SSRIs: adults and children*, the TGA cited Hall et al. (2003) as evidence that 'increased prescribing of antidepressants in Australia during 1991-2000 was associated with decreasing suicide rates.'[126] As explained above, this was wrong. Even Hall et al. stated (in the body of their article) that 'The total suicide rate for Australian men and women did not change between 1991 and 2000 because marked decreases in older men and women were offset by increases in younger adults, especially younger men'. [127] In *Suicidality with SSRIs: adults and children*, the TGA identified that there was a decrease in the suicide rate among older Australians, but did not acknowledge the more than offsetting increase in suicide by younger Australians. Although the TGA stated that Hall et al. did 'not demonstrate a causal relationship', it reinforced the suggestion that increasing SSRI prescribing rates may be 'indicative of improved overall management of depression'.[128]

It appears likely that the TGA accepted the misleading conclusion in Hall et al.'s abstract, without adequately considering the contradictory information in the body of the paper. The TGA should have done its job properly. However, if the authors of Hall et al 2003 including Hickie had written an abstract that reflected reality, perhaps the TGA may have responded more appropriately to the FDA's warning.

In 2016 – eleven years after the TGA issued its original inept response to the FDA warning – the TGA issued a *Medicines Safety Update* highlighting concerns about SSRIs and suicidality in children and adolescents.[129] It discussed research that found patients and carers were very often not informed about the potential risks of antidepressants, including suicidality risks. Had the TGA responded competently and publicly when the FDA issued its warning in 2004, it is very likely that more patients and parents would have been aware of the risk and some would have avoided taking antidepressants. Of course we can never know for sure, but it may be that some young Australians who suicided while using or withdrawing from antidepressants would be alive today if the TGA had done its job more assertively and competently 15 years ago.

GPs – Specialists in Life?

While they are clearly influential, it would be inaccurate to attribute responsibility for the rise in Australia's youth antidepressant prescribing rates to the TGA, or to a few key opinion leaders and organisations, or even the psychiatric profession alone. Most antidepressants are prescribed by general practitioners (GPs). For example, in 2014-15 (the year ending 30 June 2015), GPs prescribed 90.4% of the antidepressants prescribed to Australians of all ages. Psychiatrists were directly responsible for only 6.5%. [130] Some of the prescriptions by GPs would be repeat prescriptions for treatments initiated by psychiatrists, so the proportion initiated by GPs would be lower than 90.4%. Nonetheless, GPs clearly play a dominant role in the prescription of antidepressants in Australia.

In a 2019 TV advertising campaign GPs were marketed to Australian consumers as *Specialists in Life.* [131] In reality most are experts in 15-minute consultations [132] with at least one medication [133] as the likely outcome. Many GPs simply do not have the time or the skills needed to treat individuals distressed by grief, family breakup, unemployment or any other of life's inevitable trials. Too often a GPs only tool to deal quickly with emotionally disturbed patients are antidepressants, and if all you have is a hammer, everything looks like a nail.

How many patients (or in the case of children, parents), are informed of the risks of antidepressants by their GP, and whether their GP explores other options, and monitors their response to medication, are important unresolved questions. GPs can refer patients to a psychologist for up to twenty visits (ten individual and ten group sessions) a year under the Better Access program. But clearly with 1 in 8 Australians prescribed an antidepressant and the vast majority of prescribing done by GPs, drugs rather than Better Access psychological services are the frontline service.

In fairness to GPs, many patients do not believe that a consultation is value for both time and money if a drug or other tangible treatment does not result. In the eyes of these patients, a doctor who recommends watchful waiting, exercise, other lifestyle changes, or a visit to a psychologist, and does not produce a diagnosis and treatment, is not doing their job. This reinforces the dominance of the medical model.

Evidence that some senior GPs believe that antidepressant use prevents suicide in the general population came from an April 2019 radio interview with the President of the Royal College of General Practitioners, Dr Harry Nespolon.[134] He was being interviewed in response to media coverage of revelations that approximately 1 in 8 (over 3 million) Australians were dispensed on antidepressants in 2018 and that the vast majority of antidepressant prescribing was done by GPs.[135] Nespolon reiterated one of the most wildly inaccurate claims in the depression/suicide discourse: 'You're looking at about 1 in 6 people with untreated depression committing suicide'. Nespolon may have copied the claim from Hickie, who in 2001, while CEO of beyondblue, claimed 'people with depression have a one in six chance of being dead by suicide'.[136] Regardless of the source of his belief, claiming that 1 in 6 people with depression (either treated or untreated) die from suicide is just wrong. Irrespective of the relative risks of medication, other treatments, or no treatment, the risk of suicide associated with depression is much lower than 1 in 6.[137] [138]

This grossly inaccurate but persistent claim is likely to have emanated from the 15% suicide rate found in studies from the 1970s and earlier decades of people with treated depression, many of whom had received long-term intensive treatment including antidepressants. Diagnostic criteria for depression were much stricter when these studies were conducted, so these patients are not representative of the broader spectrum of people currently diagnosed with depression.[139]

In 1998, US researchers used a Washington State insurance database to examine the validity of the 15% suicide rate claim. The study found that the suicide risk for those treated with depression was many times lower than the 15% estimate and was lowest for patients who were not taking antidepressants:

> Risk per 100,000 person-years declined from 224 [0.22%] among patients who received any inpatient psychiatric treatment to 64 [0.06%] among those who received outpatient specialty mental health treatment to 43 [0.04%] among those treated with antidepressant medications in primary care to 0 among those treated in primary care without antidepressants.[140]

Even if these rates are converted to lifetime risk rates, they indicate not only a much, much lower risk than 1 in 6. They also suggest that antidepressant treatment increases the suicide risk.

A decade on: What does Australian 'real world' evidence tell us?

There is now nearly a decade of real-world Australian data since the Orygen/headspace Evidence Summary and the Suicide Prevention Australia position statement were published and Hickie made his unequivocal assertion that the 'real harm… comes from not receiving a diagnosis or treatment.'[141] The trends are worrying. Multiple sources, including Orygen[142], have identified rising child, adolescent and young adult antidepressant prescribing rates[143 144] and/or increasing rates of suicide[145] and self-harm[146] by young Australians over the last decade. However, the possibility that there is a link between these trends has been ignored.

Hickie and the other co-authors of Hall et al (2003) had conducted their deeply flawed analysis of 1990's data but it wasn't until in June 2019 that the first robust exploration of Australian population-based evidence on the possible link between antidepressant use and youth suicide occurred. A *PsychWatch Australia* blog I and Dr Melissa Raven wrote titled *More young Australians suicide/self-harm and use antidepressants while experts dismiss FDA warning* covered most of the issues discussed in this chapter.[147] We identified a sharp rise in both antidepressant use and suicide rates by young Australians over the preceding decade and reported that:

> 'beginning in 2008-09, an increase of approximately 60% in per-capita antidepressant use rates by young Australians (aged 0 to 27) has been associated with a 40% increase in per-capita suicide rates by young Australians (aged 0 to 24)'".[148]

Following the publication of our blog Raven and I, together with Professor Jon Jureidini, converted the blog into a peer reviewed article published in *Frontiers in Psychiatry.*[149] We collected another year's data and found that from 2008 to 2018 Australian per-capita child, adolescent and young adult antidepressant dispensing (0–27 years of age) and suicide (0–24 years) rates increased approximately 66% and 49%, respectively. Our paper's conclusion states:

> Correlation does not prove causation, and many factors impact suicide rates. However, given that the FDA warned that antidepressants were associated with an approximately doubled risk of suicidality relative to placebo, we are not surprised that rising dispensing rates have been accompanied by increasing youth suicide rates.

> In the Australian debate following the FDA warning, there were isolated voices, including the three authors of this paper, two as

researchers[150] and one as a parliamentarian[151], concerned about the effect of increasing antidepressant use on youth suicide rates. Yet these voices had little impact and, Australia-wide, there appears to have been a culture of uncritical groupthink about the relationship between treatment and youth suicide.

The dominant message in the public discourse has been that depression is very common and is serious but easily treated if only troubled young people would seek help.[152] Many who propagate this message are undoubtedly well-meaning, but the reality for too many young people is that 'help' is nothing more than a short consultation with a GP, a script for an antidepressant, and perhaps a few words of caution about possible side-effects.

Causal relationships cannot be established with certainty until there is a vast improvement in post-marketing surveillance (adverse event monitoring). However, there is clear evidence that more young Australians are taking antidepressants, and more young Australians are killing themselves and self-harming, often by intentionally overdosing on the very substances that are supposed to help them.[153]

As stated above the increase in youth antidepressant use over the last decade was predicted by myself and others. In the lead-up to the August 2010 Federal election, political activist group *GetUp* had organised candle-light vigils to highlight concerns about youth suicide. McGorry who was the serving Australian of the Year addressed these vigils.[154]

A year later I told the Western Australian Parliament that if we followed the advice of Orygen's, headspace's and McGorry's advice we should expect an 'increase in the number of candles' at the next vigil.[155] As demonstrated in the graph below this is exactly what has happened.

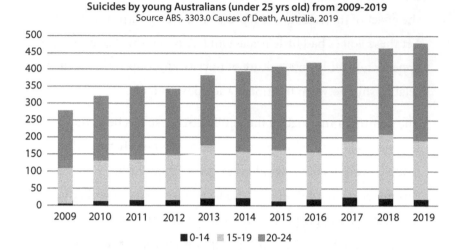

Suicides by young Australians (under 25 yrs old) from 2009-2019
Source ABS, 3303.0 Causes of Death, Australia, 2019

0-14 ■ 15-19 ■ 20-24

The above graph doesn't take account of the increase in population. Nonetheless, if the per-capita rate of under-25-year-old suicide had remained at the average rate for 2008 and 2009 levels, approximately 900 fewer young Australians would have killed themselves between 2010 and 2019.[156]

In the period immediately following the FDA issuing its initial 2004 warning, there was a large decrease in the per-capita prescribing rate to young Australians. From the year ending 30 June 2004 to the year ending 30 June 2008 the per-capita rate for Australians aged 0 to 27 years decreased steadily by a total of 32%. During this period Australia's under-25-year-olds' per-capita suicide rates was more volatile, with a weak but inconsistent downward trend.[157]

However beginning in 2009 and coinciding with the advice offered by Australia's leading suicide prevention experts – including Suicide Prevention Australia, headspace, Orygen and Professors McGorry and Hickie – antidepressant use rates began rising. This suggests it is likely that this advice contributed to the increasing antidepressant use, and thereby may have contributed to rising suicide rates among young Australians.

Not surprisingly, many suicide prevention experts seem reluctant to consider the possibility that their advice has contributed to the avoidable deaths of young Australians. Instead, they tend to hypothesise alternative explanations for rising youth suicide rates. For example, in 2016, Orygen, in collaboration with eleven other organisations (including beyondblue, the Black Dog Institute and headspace), produced a report titled *Raising the bar for youth suicide prevention*.[158] The report unambiguously identified that youth and child suicide and self-harm rates were rising, stating:

> Over the past 10 years, rather than making inroads into reducing the number of young lives lost to suicide in Australia, there have instead been small but gradual increases in suicide rates... This has mirrored high rates of self-harm among young people.[159] (p. 7)

The report hypothesised multiple possible causes including the increased use of social media, homophobia and untreated mental illness. In the entire 57-page report, the word 'medication' was mentioned once, and antidepressants and SSRIs were not mentioned at all. The highly plausible hypothesis that, in line with the FDA warning, rising antidepressant use rates are at least in part responsible for rising youth and child suicide rates, was completely ignored.

Self-Harm

There is also strong evidence that antidepressants are commonly used in self-poisoning (overdose). Research published in 2019 found 'a concerning increase in child/adolescent [aged 5 to 19 years] self-poisoning in Australia' that corresponded to an increase in psychotropic prescribing rates, particularly SSRI antidepressants. It also found that there was 'substantial overlap between the most dispensed psychotropics and medicines most commonly used in self-poisoning episodes'.[160]

Detail of Cairns et al.'s 2019 research on antidepressant use and self-harm

Cairns et al. presented evidence of increasing antidepressant prescribing rates from 2009 to 2016 in two timeframes. They cited prior research161 showing that from 2009 to 2012 antidepressant use by Australians under the age of 25 increased by 25%, and among this group grew fastest in children aged 10-14 (35.5%). They also found that, from July 2012 to June 2016, the number of individuals dispensed SSRIs increased 40% and 35% in those aged 5-14 and 15-19, respectively.

They then reviewed data from 2006 to 2016 for New South Wales and Victorian self-poisonings and found, in the under-20 age group, an increase in intentional annual poisonings of 98% from 2006 to 2016, with most of the growth occurring after 2011.

This simultaneous increase in antidepressant use and intentional self-poisoning results are consistent with the hypothesis that antidepressants increase the risk of suicidality and self-harm in young people. Even worse, they provide compelling evidence that the antidepressants prescribed to children and adolescents are frequently the means of self-harm.

In response to this research, Professor McGorry speculated that a number of possible factors may have contributed to the rising self-harm rates among young Australians, including: 'the impact of smartphones, online bullying, and a lack of meaningful face-to-face relationships [and young people's concerns about] climate change, the casualisation of the workforce, HECs debt, financial pressures, and social and environmental changes'. He also unequivocally identified that the inability of headspace to meet growing demand causing a blow-out in waiting lists is 'part of the reason why we are seeing increases in self harm and suicidal behaviour'.[162]

So, among other factors, McGorry attributed increasing self-harm and suicidal behaviour to under-funding of headspace, without acknowledging the possibility that the off-label prescribing of antidepressants to under-18s that he, Orygen and headspace endorsed might be part of the problem. And he did all this while lobbying for more money for headspace.

Despite the appalling suicide and self-harm outcomes over the last ten to fifteen years, little seems to have change in the mindset of Australia's most prominent depression and suicide 'experts'. Both Hickie and McGorry have doubled down on their support for the use of antidepressants by young Australians. On 24 June 2019, *The West Australian* newspaper published a series of articles including a front page story about a seven year old girl who became suicidal on a cocktail of psychotropic drugs including antidepressants. An article titled *It's time to rethink kids pills*[163] quoted the following excerpt from a letter I wrote to Prime Minister Scott Morrison:

> Over the last decade Australian psychiatric practice, much of which is conducted by GPs with little training, has substantially ignored the FDA and TGA's warnings and followed advice of local 'experts'. The results are that over the last decade the 0 to 27-year-old prescribing rate per capita has risen about 60 per cent, (while) 0 to 24-year-old per capita suicide rates have risen 40 per cent.[164] [Note: an extra year of data has become available since then, demonstrating an estimated 66% increase in antidepressant use and an actual 49% increase in the suicide rate.]

In response Professor Patrick McGorry said that the association made between increased antidepressant use and suicide rates simply did 'not hold up…Antidepressants do not increase suicide. Evidence shows there can be a temporary increase in suicidal ideation …. (but) they reduce suicide risk in most'. By pure coincidence on the same day

McGorry's comment were reported a study was published that reviewed the information on antidepressant trials held by the FDA and found that 'the rate of suicide [attempts and completed suicides] was about 2.5 times higher in antidepressant arms relative to placebo'.[165]

Professor Hickie was also quoted in *The West Australian* article as saying:

They (critics) are acting like there's something wrong with increasing treatment…As treatment goes up, we have to be careful, we do run the danger as we increase access…that the trade-off is low-quality care. But what's the alternative? No care?

The obvious response to Professor Hickie is that, when 'increasing treatment' is clearly associated with increasing death by suicide among young Australians, 'there's something wrong'. Perhaps Professor Hickie needs to ponder the meaning of 'first do no harm'?

In fairness to McGorry and Hickie, they were responding to media reporting of the details of a blog and the internet is chock full of rubbish masquerading as science. However, when this blog was converted into a peer reviewed paper published in a reputable journal it would seem reasonable to expect them to respond with more rigour. However a year later both tripled down on their position and failed to address the evidence contained within the article Raven, Jureidini and I wrote that was published in *Frontiers in Psychiatry*.[166]

The journal article attracted media and long overdue political interest. Double Walkley Award winning journalist Jill Margot wrote an article in the *Australian Financial Review* with the headline *Suicide prevention experts may have got it 'horribly wrong'*.[167] Hickie was quoted in the article:

Contrary to this implication [that experts were in part responsible for the increase in prescribing], experts in the field…advocate for psychological counselling, and medication is restricted to those who fail to respond or have other indicators that they would be likely to respond.

I obviously disagree with Hickie. I contend that in the past he and other experts have effectively endorsed antidepressants as a means of reducing suicide risk in young people and that this is likely to have contributed to Australians extraordinarily high rates of antidepressant use. However, Hickie's comment in the *Australian Financial Review* was measured and well within the boundaries of appropriate public debate.

In contrast, McGorry's responded to our peer reviewed journal article by 'spitting the dummy' on National Radio. In a very soft interview with McGorry, ABC Radio National's Drive Host, Patricia Karvelas, briefly referred to the *Australian Financial Review* article and asked McGorry what our study 'claimed to show'. He replied:

> It wasn't really a study. It was more like you know a piece of propaganda and these people have been at it for years and years… there is some grain of truth in what these people are on about but they are on a mission and I was very surprised that that paper got published and I certainly was very surprised that *AFR* ran it but …every… 6 or 12 months we have this issue about drugging our kids coming up again it's a very unsophisticated way to look at it and you know we have got around that by involving young people and involving the whole range of stakeholders in the way that this care is provided and we actually go with evidence. We don't go with polemic.[168]

McGorry is correct in that 'these people' – Raven, Jureidini and I – have 'been on a mission for years'. But our mission is to have mental health policy and practice driven by robust, independent, contestable evidence. Our paper detailed the Australian response to the FDA and TGA warnings and population outcomes in terms of suicide and self-harm rates. It included detailed referenced criticisms of the flawed evidence base McGorry and others used to justify their advice that antidepressants reduce the risk of youth suicidality. That is how scientific debate should occur. It is laughable that McGorry ended his answer with the claim that 'we don't go with polemic' having begun it by dismissing the work of those who disagree with him as 'propaganda'. He failed to address the substantive issues we (these people) raised in our paper and resorted to the 'polemic'.

Two days after McGorry was interviewed by Karvales the Sunday edition of the *Sydney Morning Herald* reported that the Morrison Government Minster for Heath Greg Hunt:

> 'Has asked his department to review the results of an academic study linking the increase in youth suicide with a rise in antidepressants being prescribed to Australian children'... A spokesman for Mr Hunt said the minister 'is deeply concerned by the rate of depression and suicide among young Australians' and that the TGA would review the Curtin study's findings 'and, if necessary, take strong and appropriate action'.[169]

The Sydney Morning Herald article also covered an impassioned and informed speech in the Australian Parliament made a week earlier by Labor MP Julian Hill who cited our paper and called on Minister Hunt to establish a national inquiry into the role of antidepressants in youth suicide. Hill told the Australian Parliament 'Correlation is not causation but, with ten years of data going in the wrong direction, we cannot continue to ignore this issue'.[170]

Hill's call for an inquiry and Hunt's positive response was very welcome. I have never doubted that the Morrison Government and previous Commonwealth Governments genuinely desire reduced suicide rates and achieve better mental health outcomes. But until this announcement every indication was that they were determined to take advice from the same experts and give more money to the same services that to date have failed so badly.

After his surprise victory in the May 2019 Federal Election Prime Minister Scott Morrison declared tackling suicide was one of his Government's top priorities. Health Minister Greg Hunt immediately convened an emergency meeting of Australia's 'leading mental health experts' including Professors McGorry and Hickie. The outcome of the Melbourne meeting was that the Federal Government announced it was considering establishing *junior headspace* targeting children aged five to 11. After the roundtable Professor McGorry told *The West Australian* 'We need integrated care centres that are tailored for different age groups, including very young children'. Professor Hickie told *The West Australian* the roundtable agreed that the deficit in child mental health services could not continue.[171]

In a similar vein in the lead up to the May 2019 Federal Election Morrison's Liberal Party had announced its $503.1 million *Youth Mental Health and Suicide Prevention Plan* which it declared was 'the largest suicide prevention strategy in Australia's history'.[172] The lion's share of the money – $375million – was allocated to 'expand and improve the headspace network'.[173]

A few weeks after the roundtable I wrote an open letter to Prime Minister Morrison and Health Minister Greg Hunt pleading 'Re: youth suicide and antidepressants. Please don't listen to the same failed local experts'.[174] In the letter I detailed the history of the FDA and TGA warnings and the response by Professors McGorry and Hickie and headspace, Orygen and Suicide Prevention Australia and the subsequent upward spiral in antidepressant use and youth suicide. I pointed out that I had predicted this in 2011 and concluded:

> I take no satisfaction in being proved correct. I am frustrated and angry that the same voices pushing the same failed programs still dominate the national debate about youth suicide prevention, despite their very poor track record. To put it bluntly, I strongly

contend that without change, it is likely that antidepressant use and suicide rates among young Australians will continues to increase.

Minister Hunt responded on behalf of the Morrison Government. His letter did not address the impact of the advice provided by headspace, Orygen, Professor McGorry, Professor Hickie and *Suicide Prevention Australia*. It made no reference to the positive correlation between increasing suicide rates and antidepressant use and self-harm rates among young Australians since these failed suicide prevention experts offered their advice.[175]

I was very disappointed with Minister Hunt's response. To me he seemed incapable of acknowledging these facts and past policy failures – even when the other side of politics was in charge. Instead he appeared to be charmed and bamboozled by mental health entrepreneurs promising 21st century solutions to problems that the evidence indicates they have helped create.

However, in fairness to Minister Hunt he was responding to a letter from a private citizen (me) who has no medical training that was critical of prominent mental health organisations and generally well-respected professors of psychiatry. When he responded to Hill's call he was responding to a Member of Parliament and a peer reviewed article in a respected journal. The information in both my letter and the journal article may have been substantially the same but the context was very different.

I was very pleased when Minister Hunt initiated the review of the issues raised in our *Frontiers in Psychiatry* paper. At last it brought hope of an open debate about the relationship between antidepressant use and youth suicide, and perhaps more broadly about the safety and efficacy of other mental health interventions.

I was even more pleased when the TGA released its review findings in mid-December 2020. Like our research it found a correlation between antidepressant use and suicide among Australians aged under 25 years. It quite correctly concluded (as we had) that the "current evidence available is insufficient to conclude that a causal relationship exists" but committed the TGA to immediately:

> Explore potential analysis of linked PBS, Medicare Benefits Schedule (MBS), hospital and death data to further investigate the clinical journeys of young people prescribed antidepressants in Australia and the relationship between antidepressants and rates of youth suicide. In addition there will be consideration of the utility of established datasets held by the Australian Bureau of Statistics and the Australian Institute of Health and Welfare.

This sort of analysis, if done properly, could move our understanding of the relationship between antidepressant use and youth suicide beyond correlation, to something more definitive. The TGA should have done this sort of post market analysis years ago, however it is always better late than never!

The current administration of the TGA, Health Minister Greg Hunt and Julian Hill MP deserve credit. Thankfully, at last they have ended the era of wilful blindness to the real possibility that antidepressants may be part of the problem, not the solution.

Chapter 5

Patrick McGorry's Ultra-High Risk Crusade

Patrick McGorry is Professor of Youth Mental Health at the University of Melbourne. He has authored or co-authored over 900 'scholarly works'.[176] He is the Executive Director of Orygen, The National Centre of Excellence in Youth Mental Health and founding editor of *Early Intervention in Psychiatry*, published by the International Early Psychosis Association.[177] McGorry also advocated strongly for the establishment of the Australian government funded National Youth Mental Health Foundation, which became headspace, and he is a founding board member[178]. McGorry played a central role in designing and advocating for the scaling up of headspace services. In 2010 he was awarded Australian of the Year. Both McGorry and organisations he has led, particularly earlier in his career, have received financial support from multiple pharmaceutical companies.

Professor McGorry is arguably the world's most prominent advocate of Preventive Psychiatry. He has an unshakable belief that, prior to the onset of psychosis, depression and other serious mental illnesses, there is a 'prodromal phase' and that intervening then will help save many the misery of full-blown mental illness. McGorry's Preventive Psychiatry 'stitch in time' theories are intuitively appealing.[179] Why would you not intervene if you could prevent mental illness?

The problem is you can't. Despite nearly thirty years of trying, McGorry's version of Preventive Psychiatry simply does not work. Clinicians cannot predict with sufficient accuracy who will go on to become ill; and even when they do get it right, the preventive measures simply do not have sustained long-term benefits. Even McGorry has acknowledged that the vast majority of people that are identified as being at ultra-high risk of developing psychosis, one of his specialist areas, never become psychotic.

McGorry describes his approach as 'Early Intervention', but in reality it often involves intervening earlier than early. It involves intervening in cases where most patients, left untreated, will never become mentally ill. The massive false positive rate is a real negative of Preventive Psychiatry. Adding to this concern is McGorry's long history of unsuccessfully experimenting with psychotropic drugs as a means of saving people considered at elevated risk of future mental illness.

Decades of failure have not curbed McGorry's infectious enthusiasm, and his impressive marketing and lobbying skills have made the philosophy of preventive psychiatry massively influential in Australia. Every Australia Government, from the Gillard Government in 2010 to the Morrison Government in 2020, has committed hundreds of millions of dollars to McGorry's pet projects like headspace and Early Psychosis Prevention and Intervention Centres (EPPIC). This is despite a dearth of robust, independent evidence that any of this actually helps. It is not surprising to those of us who have watched this debacle unfold that the results – unlike the rhetoric – have been so alarmingly uninspiring.

McGorry may choose other words, but the essence of his prodromal theory is that agitation, distress and anxiety are frequently indicators that adolescents and young adults are very likely to experience full-blown mental illness. He believes that intervening in this prodromal phase will help save many young people from avoidable misery and suffering. Much of McGorry's prodromal theorising relates to psychosis. He believes that behaviours like occasionally struggling to find an appropriate word, or being occasionally concerned that other are gossiping about them, are tell-tale signs that a young person is at 'ultra-high risk' of becoming psychotic.[180]

The term 'ultra-high risk' implies that it is very likely that the potential psychiatric patient will transition from distress to disease. It is an alarming, potentially stigmatising and completely misleading label. Credible evidence shows the conversion rate for those considered at ultra-high risk to first episode psychosis may be as low as 8%.[181] Even headspace has acknowledged that 82% to 90% of the people identified as being at ultra-high risk of developing psychosis do not become psychotic within a year.[182] However, both McGorry and headspace[183] argue that the use of the term is justified because the likelihood of them becoming psychotic is considerably higher than that of the general population.

They are correct in that anxious, distressed teenagers and young adults have a higher risk of future psychosis than their peers. But with a 90%+ false positive rate, the real ultra-high risk is the near certainty of being incorrectly labelled as being 'pre-psychotic' – a term McGorry has used interchangeably with 'prodromal' and 'ultra-high risk'.[184]

It is also important to note that 'psychotic symptoms in teenagers are often transient, caused by substance abuse or mood disorder'.[185] While working as a mental health advocate, I supported a number of young Australians desperate to lose the schizophrenic label they had been given as a result of a single psychotic episode resulting from drug use. Teenagers and young adults should have the right to run off the rails and then get back on track without some overconfident diagnostician applying a stigmatising label that is near impossible to shake off. The ultra-high risk diagnosis extends the risk of applying stigmatising labels to those who are mildly distressed, but have never actually lost the plot.

I attended a conference in Perth in 2012 where Professor McGorry was a member of a panel of mental health experts. Another guest expert, American psychologist Professor Gail Horstein, said the single biggest lesson she had learned in 30 years in the field was that psychiatric labels often become stigmatising self-fulfilling prophecies. In response, McGorry did what I have seen him do on numerous occasions. He gave the impression he agreed with the previous speaker and thereby avoided confrontation. He told the audience, which included many self-described 'psychiatric survivors', that he too was very concerned about the potential for labels to become self-fulfilling prophecies.

In a Q&A that followed, I asked McGorry to reconcile those concerns with his use of the term 'ultra-high risk' and the fact that, by his own admission, the vast majority of those who get the label will never become psychotic. I said the normal 'non-expert' patient and family interpretation of the term ultra-high risk would be that future psychosis was probable rather than possible and that the term was misleading and stigmatising and should be dropped.

Professor McGorry, with charm and grace, accepted my point both in the forum and again in a brief private discussion we had outside the forum. McGorry had told me what I wanted to hear. He left me thinking that the term ultra-high risk would be changed and replaced with something more accurate and less alarming (e.g. increased or elevated risk).

That was over seven years ago, and there has been no change. In 2019, McGorry reiterated his belief that the ultra-high risk diagnosis pioneered at Orygen, 'has been tremendously useful for detecting those at risk of developing schizophrenia and other psychotic disorders'.[186]

I doubt McGorry's capacity to respond to contradictory evidence. However, I have no doubt that he is motivated by a burning desire to help young Australians. He has a crusader's zeal and is determined to do what he is convinced are great works regardless of all obstacles in his path. Professor Allen Frances, who was also a panellist at the conference, had earlier reached a similar conclusion, writing:

> McGorry's intentions are clearly noble, but so were Don Quixote's. The kindly knight's delusional good intentions and misguided interventions wreaked havoc and confusion at every turn. Sad to say, Australia's well intended impulse to protect its children will paradoxically put them at greater risk. Let's applaud McGorry's vision but not blindly follow him down an unknown path fraught with dangers.[187]

Few people have the time or inclination to scrutinise details of Professor McGorry's work. His theory that psychosis can be spotted and prevented before it occurs is intuitively appealing. However, he has so much invested in this theory that he is unable to accept the independent evidence that it cannot be reliably predicted and that pre-intervention (prevention) simply does not work. Frances was correct, Australia should never have let McGorry's enthusiasm, however admirable and infectious, trump the evidence and drive the direction of national mental health policy.

I also agree with Frances that McGorry may ultimately have noble intentions but he is no Don Quixote. He is shrewd, he is smart and he knows what it takes to win the hearts, minds and approval of those that matter. He is easily the most effective lobbyist, marketer and political operator I have encountered.

McGorry, Psychosis Risk Disorder and DSM-5

The debate about the proposed recognition of a new psychiatric disorder,

Attenuated Psychosis Syndrome, commonly known as Psychosis Risk Disorder, in the DSM-5, revealed much about the way McGorry operates.

As detailed in Chapters 2 and 3, Australian psychiatric practice typically follows American psychiatry's DSM lead. Early drafts of DSM-5 included a new disorder – Attenuated Psychosis Syndrome – commonly known as Psychosis Risk Disorder. Its inclusion in the final version of DSM-5 published in 2013 would have classified young Australians, deemed to be at ultra-high risk of psychosis, as having a psychiatric disorder requiring treatment.

The planned inclusion received widespread international criticism led by Frances. He nominated, Psychosis Risk Syndrome as 'the most ill-conceived and potentially harmful' of all the proposals for insertion into DSM-5.

> The whole concept of early intervention rests on three fundamental [flawed] pillars … 1) it would misidentify many teenagers who are not really at risk for psychosis; 2) the treatment they would most often receive (atypical antipsychotic medication) has no proven efficacy; but, 3) it does have definite dangerous complications.[188]

On the other side of the Atlantic Til Wykes, Professor of Clinical Psychology and Rehabilitation at King's College London, expressed similar concerns. In 2011, she co-authored an editorial in the *Journal of Mental Health* claiming the concept was not based on sound evidence and highlighting the dangers of stigma and unnecessary harmful treatments. 'It is a bit like telling ten people with the common cold that they are 'at risk for pneumonia syndrome' when only one is likely to get the disorder'.[189]

Mercifully, in May 2011, the American Psychiatric Association's DSM-5 task force revealed the group decided not to include Attenuated Psychosis Syndrome because of concerns that 'this diagnosis might result in inappropriate treatments'.[190]

A year earlier, in May 2010, before the backlash against Psychosis Risk Disorder got significant Australian media coverage, McGorry was quoted in an article in the *Psychiatry Update* titled *DSMV [DSM-5] 'risk syndrome': a good start, should go further*. He said 'the proposal for DSMV to include a "risk syndrome" reflecting an increased likelihood of mental illness is welcome but does not go far enough'.[191]

In a similar vein, a few months earlier, McGorry had written a journal article, titled *New diagnostic infrastructure for early intervention in psychiatry*, which concluded:

> The proposal to consider including the concept of the risk syndrome in the forthcoming revision of the DSM classification is innovative and timely. It has not come out of left field, however, and is based upon a series of conceptual and empirical foundations built over the past 15 years.[192]

Soon after McGorry made his confident assertions, the debate started to change. There was significant media coverage critical of the idea of including Psychosis Risk Disorder in DSM-5. In May 2011 Professor McGorry and I were interviewed separately by ABC Radio's *World Today* program. I described McGorry as a leading international proponent of Psychosis Risk Syndrome's inclusion in the next edition of DSM. McGorry responded by saying, 'contrary to Mr Whitely's statements, I haven't been pushing for it to be included in DSM-5. Now that hasn't been my position. But it's a new area of work. It's only been studied for the last 15 years'.[193] McGorry also told the *Monthly* that he did not mind if the syndrome is included in the manual or not, but he 'won't resile from the fact that we were the ones to [develop] the idea and it has been a major advance in psychiatry'.[194]

So within a year, McGorry had gone from arguing the proposal to put Attenuated Psychosis Syndrome (Psychosis Risk Disorder) in the DSM-5 as 'innovative and timely... based on 15 years of empirical evidence...

but does not go far enough' to 'I haven't been pushing for it... It's only been studied for the last 15 years'.

The hypocrisy was obvious; however, I did not criticise him for this at the time. McGorry and I had met at Parliament House in Perth, and we were engaged in polite and what I thought at the time were positive discussions. I thought it wise to let him back down with dignity.

I was even more encouraged in February 2012 when McGorry acknowledged the widespread international concern with the inclusion of Psychosis Risk Disorder in DSM-5 and told the *Sydney Morning Herald* that he now opposed its inclusion.[195] I subsequently wrote a blog titled *Patrick McGorry deserves praise for about-turn on Psychosis Risk Disorder*.[196] I was prepared to forget his prior duplicity; however, it later became obvious that McGorry had not changed his position.

McGorry on the use of antipsychotics to prevent psychosis

Prior to the DSM-5 Psychosis Risk debate, McGorry had enthusiastically promoted the potential of antipsychotics to prevent psychosis. Three examples include:

1. In 2006, McGorry was the lead author of an article which, as part of a proposed 'clinical staging framework', identified 'atypical antipsychotic agents', as one of the 'potential interventions' for individuals who are at 'ultra-high risk (10% to 40%)' of developing first episode psychosis.[197]

2. In a 2007 article, *Prediction of psychosis: setting the stage*, jointly authored by Professor McGorry and Associate Professor Alison Yung stated results of trials 'suggest that both antipsychotic medication and psychological interventions might have a role in treating the difficulties and problems young people at ultra-high risk experience as well as delaying or preventing the onset of psychosis'.[198] Their paper began by quoting a 1994 paper (Mrazek & Haggerty[199]) extolling the

potential of pre-psychosis pharmacological interventions:

> The best hope now for the prevention of schizophrenia lies
> with indicated preventive interventions targeted at individuals
> manifesting precursor signs and symptoms who have not yet met
> full criteria for diagnosis. The identification of individuals at this
> early stage, coupled with the introduction of pharmacological and
> psychosocial interventions, may prevent the development of the
> full-blown disorder.

McGorry's article's opening comment followed: 'Such sentiment underlines the aim of people in the prodromal phase preceding a first psychotic episode'. The article went on to outline evidence supporting interventions including antipsychotics 'to delay or even prevent onset of psychosis'.[200]

3. In 2008, in a *British Medical Journal* article titled *'Is early intervention in the major psychiatric disorders justified? Yes'*, McGorry wrote:

> Early intervention covers both early detection and the phase
> specific treatment of the earlier stages of illness with psychosocial
> and drug interventions. It should be as central in psychiatry as
> it is in cancer, diabetes, and cardiovascular disease… Several
> randomised controlled trials have shown that it is possible
> to delay the onset of fully fledged psychotic illness in young
> people at very high risk of early transition with either low dose
> antipsychotic drugs or cognitive behavioural therapy.[201]

Despite this early enthusiasm, later in the face of growing criticism of the DMS-5 Psychosis Risk Disorder proposal and his advocacy of the use of antipsychotics to prevent psychosis, McGorry changed his tone. In December 2010, he wrote *'Antipsychotic medications should not be considered unless there is a clear-cut and sustained progression to frank psychotic disorder meeting full DSM 4 criteria.'* He then immediately invalidated this statement, writing:

The only exception to the previous statement is where there has been a definite failure to respond to the first and second line interventions described above AND there is worsening and continuing disability, or significant risk of self-harm, suicide or harm to others arising directly from the **mental disorder itself** and its symptoms. In this situation, a trial of low dose antipsychotic medication for 6 weeks in the first instance may be appropriate, with careful monitoring for adverse events.[202]

The words 'mental disorder itself' are revealing. McGorry must have been referring to Psychosis Risk Syndrome, which was not at the time a recognised psychiatric disorder (and hopefully never will be).

In May 2011, when facing significant critical scrutiny, McGorry wrote 'our clinical guidelines do not (and have never done so in the past) recommend the use of anti-psychotic medication as the first line or standard treatment for this ultra-high risk group'.[203] While they may not have been formally endorsed, final 'clinical guidelines', as previously outlined, for well over a decade, McGorry had advocated the likely benefits of the pre-emptive prescription of antipsychotics to adolescents at ultra-high risk of psychosis.

Three months later, it became obvious that his core belief that antipsychotics may help prevent psychosis had not changed. In August 2011, *The Sunday Age* newspaper, in an article titled *Drug trial scrapped amid outcry,* reported how 'Patrick McGorry has aborted a controversial trial of antipsychotic drugs on children as young as 15 who are "at risk" of psychosis, amid complaints the study was unethical'.[204] *The Sunday Age* revealed that 13 researchers from Australia, Britain and America had lodged a formal complaint calling for the NEURAPRO-Q trial not to go ahead. They were concerned children who had not yet been diagnosed with a psychotic illness would be unnecessarily given drugs with potentially dangerous side effects.

McGorry told the *Sunday Age* the decision to scrap the trial was made in June 2011 and was unrelated to the complaint. He said the trial was abandoned due to 'feasibility issues' with recruiting participants in Europe and America. It was reported that McGorry 'acknowledged the evidence suggested antipsychotics were not effective as a first-line treatment for the at-risk group' but 'he would consider a similar trial on patients for whom other treatments had failed'.[205] McGorry also told the *Sunday Age* that concerns that the clinical services he leads might eventually medicate at-risk young people were unfounded.

There has been little (if any) independent public scrutiny of headspace and headspace-run Early Psychosis Service prescribing practices, so it is not known if antipsychotics are prescribed to prevent psychosis at these services or elsewhere in Australia. However, the idea that antipsychotics may help prevent psychosis – espoused by McGorry and his colleagues – has been influential internationally. Recent research published in the *Australian and New Zealand Journal of Psychiatry* revealed that the practice of using antipsychotics among those considered to be at elevated risk of psychosis is 'widely practiced' in China but does not work.

The research, first published in May 2020, followed the outcomes of 450 'individuals with a clinical high risk (CHR) of psychosis' for three years. Of these, 319 were treated with antipsychotics and 141 were not. The researchers found:

> Patients who did not receive antipsychotics showed a lower conversion rate than those who did... In mild CHR cases, antipsychotic treatment was more likely to be associated with conversion to psychosis, compared with the no-antipsychotics group, with no such difference observed in severe CHR cases. Among those who received antipsychotics, monotherapy or low-dose treatment was associated with lower conversion rates.[206]

The researchers concluded 'administration of antipsychotics to CHR patients is potentially harmful with no preventive benefits'.

This research should have ended McGorry's thirty-year quest for drugs to be used as a preventive treatment. But it didn't. In September 2020, it was announced with great fanfare that Orygen had secured $33 million, the largest ever Australian mental health research grant from a foreign funding source. The money, from the US National Institutes for Health, is to be used to breathe new life into McGorry's three-decade-long quest to develop a reliable and safe way of identifying young people who are at 'imminent and high' risk of becoming psychotic.[207] The hope is that Orygen will develop better 'prediction models' to enable the achievement of 'a holy grail in this area - more effective preventive treatments tailored to individual patients'.[208]

The project - *Trajectories and Predictors in the Clinical High Risk for Psychosis population: Australian Network of Clinics and international Partners* - is part of a bigger $82 million US-led Accelerating Medicines [Schizophrenia Research] Partnership that includes multiple drug companies as partners.[209] [210] According to McGorry, the overall aim of the partnership is to 'provide a pathway to a more targeted drug discovery, because that is what we really need to get much better outcomes for these illnesses'.[211]

If the trial goes ahead, Orygen will recruit approximately a thousand young people they judge to be at high risk of psychosis, and will undertake 'a range of assessments – clinical interviews, neurocognitive and neurophysiological assessments, brain imaging and genetics'.[212] [213]

In an interview with a senior ABC journalist, Fran Kelly, McGorry said:

> We've already developed good psycho-social treatments for this stage of illness which are quite effective, but we do need safer and more effective biological therapies. I have been measuring bio markers of various kinds including imaging and a whole range of

blood bio markers as well which we know are actually associated with the onset of the illness too.[214]

McGorry's statement invited the following three obvious follow up questions, but Kelly failed to ask any of them:

1.   Most of those identified by you and Orygen in your prior research as being at ultra-high risk never become psychotic. Isn't it misleading to describe them as being at a 'stage of illness'?

2.   If as you claim, Orygen has already developed 'good, effective psycho-social treatments' for the ultra-high risk group, why do these young people need drug treatment when less invasive and potentially harmful treatments exist?

3.   Despite decades of well-funded research, there are no diagnostic biomarkers for any mainstream psychiatric disorder, but you appear to be saying you have found biomarkers that are indicative of schizophrenia in people who have never been psychotic. How can this be?

As happens far too often, an ABC journalist failed to challenge McGorry (especially his extraordinary biomarker claim). Instead, the ABC acted like McGorry and Orygen's advertorial channel. Hardly behaviour we should accept from our generally respected, publicly funded broadcaster (see Chapter 8).

While the $33 million Australian leg of the ongoing $82 million US-led Partnership does not currently involve experimenting with drugs, it lays the groundwork for future drug trials, with approximately a thousand distressed young Australians likely to be given the stigmatising ultra-high-risk label.

Surely three decades of failure is enough to accept that the concept is fundamentally flawed? But no, not for McGorry, Orygen and their international partners – which include numerous drug companies. They are obviously determined to have another go at promoting the ultra-high risk/psychosis risk disorder/attenuated psychosis syndrome label, and finding drugs to match.

The History of EPPIC and EPYS

In 2005, Orygen Youth Health, led by McGorry, opened an EPPIC (Early Psychosis Prevention and Intervention Centre) in North West Melbourne 'resourced to help just 250 young people each year'.[215] In 2006, the first headspace was opened with $54 million in Australian Government funding.[216] By 2020, McGorry had driven the establishment of 14 Early Psychosis Youth Services (EPYS)[217] located within some of the over 130 headspace services[218] across Australia.

Over those 15 years – which have been the most chaotic in Australian political history –McGorry and colleagues have endured many threats to the funding of Early Psychosis Services and headspace. McGorry has successfully lobbied seven Prime Ministers from both sides of Australian politics to achieve bipartisan support for expanding EPPIC and headspace. However, his success getting state Premiers to commit resources to his pet programs has been mixed. Some – particularly Victorian Premier Daniel Andrews – have wholeheartedly embraced McGorry and his programs. Others have been less effusive in their praise and resisted committing state funds to jointly fund (with the Commonwealth Government) McGorry-inspired programs. Whether this is because they resent the Commonwealth interfering in what is a state's responsibility, and/or are concerned about duplication, or they are quietly unimpressed with the evidence supporting McGorry-inspired programs, is unclear.

McGorry's crusade to spot and eliminate psychosis in young people before it occurs received a huge boost when, in January 2010, he was announced as 2010 Australian of the Year. When presenting the award, then Prime Minister Kevin Rudd said:

The incredible influence of his work, the number of young
Australians and their families whose lives have been improved,
and the value of his contribution to the nation cannot ever fully
be measured... With this award, we recognise that we have
in Professor McGorry a leader whose drive, compassion, and
commitment to understanding and treating youth mental illness
has helped shaped not only lives, but our national approach to
mental health intervention, prevention and treatment.[219]

Perhaps Prime Minister Rudd's comment about the value of
McGorry's contribution never being fully measured were a veiled
reference to the lack of evidence supporting the hype around McGorry
and his programs. There was certainly no rigorous external analysis
supporting the marketing. Nonetheless, as the reigning Australian of the
Year, McGorry was in the national media spotlight in the lead-up to the
August 2010 Australian Commonwealth election.

A minimum of digging by the media at that time might have
tempered the adulation of McGorry by the media and all sides
of politics. He was almost universally presented as a trustworthy,
independent, authoritative, voice on mental health. This was only four
years after *Time* magazine had detailed his 'Drugs Before Diagnosis'
approach to the use of antipsychotics by non-psychotic adolescents.[220]
It was also only two years after McGorry, as an author of an article
extolling the virtues of early intervention, was required by the *BMJ* to
declare that he had received unrestricted grants from Janssen-Cilag, Eli
Lilly, Bristol Myer Squibb, Astra-Zeneca, Pfizer, and Novartis and had
acted as a paid consultant or speaker for most of these companies.[221]

When McGorry was made Australian of the Year, he was also the
Treasurer (and past President) of the *International Early Psychosis
Association,* which is funded by antipsychotic manufacturers Astra
Zeneca, Lilly and Janssen-Cilag.[222] And he was also the Director

of Clinical Services at Orygen Youth Health Clinical Program and Executive Director of the Orygen Youth Health Research Centre, which had received funding from AstraZeneca, Bristol Myer Squibb, Eli Lilly, and Janssen-Cilag.[223] All of this was missed or considered irrelevant by Australia's star-struck media and politicians.

2010 election campaign

As the reigning Australian of the Year, McGorry used the lead-up to the August 2010 election to skillfully and passionately sell his message that there was massive unmet need for services that treat mental illness among young Australians and that EPPIC and headspace should fill the void. His combination of excessive pessimism about the widespread prevalence of mental illness and optimistic promises of '21st century' solutions' – which happen to have been developed by him and his allies – was very effective.[224]

McGorry acknowledged this in March 2011, when interviewed by the *Irish Echo*, Australia's Irish Newspaper, about his advocacy as Australian of the Year before an election.

> I went into campaign mode from day one. I have a young
> Irishman called Matthew Hamilton who worked for me
> back in 2004. He's got a lot of political skill. He came out [to
> Australia] and worked for me and he's still here, he's been a
> campaign director for the whole year. We worked on it pretty
> systematically throughout the whole year. Labor were wrong-
> footed by the Opposition seizing the high moral ground but to
> their credit (following Labor's narrow victory) they have come
> back from that and they have set things up to address that,
> I have cautious optimism about Julia Gillard and especially
> [Minister for Mental Health and Ageing] Mark Butler — he has
> been an excellent minister so far. But look, if they don't get the

support from the party they are going to be in a lot of trouble with this issue again.[225]

He used the language of '21st century' solutions on multiple occasions in 2010, including in July when addressing the National Press Club[226] in the lead up to the federal election and again after the election in November when he effusively gushed about his own pet programs.

> One of the most exciting things about living in Australia today is that we have the solutions at our disposal to put such 21st century thinking into practice. We no longer need to wait for new discoveries in the health sciences – there are proven models of care available to us now.[227]

Less than a month before election-day, in a televised forum about mental health, the Labor Government was represented by the future Minister for Mental Health Mark Butler and the Liberal/National opposition by Shadow Minister Peter Dutton. Also on the panel was Professor John Mendoza, who at the time was a close ally of McGorry. McGorry's/Mendoza's blessing was desperately being sought by Dutton and Butler on behalf of their respective parties. Most enamoured of McGorry's 'early intervention' approach was Peter Dutton, who stated 'Well, we're going to roll out a national scheme based on advice by people like John Mendoza, Pat McGorry, Ian Hickey [sic], David Crosby and others… early intervention is proven without any doubt to work.'[228] Mendoza[229] reciprocated Dutton's fawning admiration, describing the Coalition's approach as 'streets ahead. It's literally comparing an old clunker to a brand new motor vehicle'. The Coalition, led by Tony Abbott, had promised to spend $1.5 billion on mental health programs, primarily focused on youth mental health.

Later in the campaign, on behalf of the Gillard Labor Government, Health Minister Nicola Roxon fought back by claiming that the Coalition's mental health plan will result in cuts elsewhere in the health sector.

'We fundamentally don't believe that it helps people with mental health issues or problems to pull money out of GP services, after-hours services, [and] e-health investments in order to fund a mental health plan'.[230] Largely due to the advocacy of McGorry and his allies, mental health was unquestionably a net positive for the Coalition in the election.

Australian politicians were keen to get McGorry's endorsement. No significant political figure has ever publicly challenged his claims of proven 21st century solutions. He claims moral and scientific authority and, because very few are prepared to challenge his claims, he achieves it.

Criticism from within the psychiatric profession are more common, but is generally polite and (ineffectually) subtle. One exception was Professor of Psychiatry at the University of New South Wales, Vaughan Carr. He wrote an opinion piece in the lead up to the 2010 election that dismissed McGorry's claim that youth-focused early psychosis intervention is 'so effective' it cuts 'costs over the longer term to one-third the usual amount' as 'a utopian fantasy' based on 'published evidence (that) is not credible'.[231] Carr's opinion piece concluded:

So this is a plea to our politicians… Let us not determine how to provide mental health care on the basis of an election-stimulated policy auction, influenced disproportionately by a vocal professional minority pushing an early intervention agenda. Mental health care is broader than that, and much too important to sell it so far short, of what it deserves.[232]

However, Carr's pull-no-punches plea fell on deaf ears. The August 2010 election result was the closest in Australian history. A minority Labor Government, led by Australia's first women Prime Minister Julia Gillard (who had deposed Kevin Rudd as PM in June 2010), was re-elected. The Gillard Government relied on the support of the Greens Party and two independent members of parliament, Tony Windsor and

Rob Oakeshott, who had previously been members of the Conservative Coalition parties.

Post 2010 election

After the election, Professor McGorry and his allies lobbied the Gillard Government to match the Coalition's 2010 election commitment of $440m to EPPIC (Early Psychosis Prevention and Intervention Centres) like those run by *Orygen Youth Health*. The minority Gillard Government could not afford to alienate prominent opinion leaders like McGorry. His momentum was irresistible, and the Government needed all the political support it could get. The Government embraced the McGorry, Hickie, Mendoza vision for Australian mental health by bringing McGorry and Hickie inside government planning processes.

A few months after the election, in December 2010, the Minister for Mental Health and Ageing, Mark Butler, took the unusual step of sidelining his own National Advisory Council on Mental Health established to give him advice on strategic directions for mental health.[233] He appointed Professors McGorry and Hickie as members of a Mental Health Expert Working Group. Minister Butler claimed the creation of this 'new, time limited, specialist group will allow for targeted advice to be provided directly to the Australian Government on how to achieve the most coordinated, cost-effective and lasting reforms for their investment in mental health care.'[234]

The Mental Health Expert Working Group was chaired by Minister Butler. The Vice Chair appointed by the Minister was Monsignor David Cappo who was previously the Social Inclusion Commissioner for the State of South Australia, while also serving as Vicar General of the Roman Catholic Archdiocese of Adelaide.

This attempt to bring these powerful mental health entrepreneurs inside government processes took an interesting twist. For reasons that are not clear, McGorry and Hickie and Monsignor David Cappo, subsequently established and led the Independent Mental Health Reform Group. In March 2011, the Independent Mental Health Reform Group released, to much media acclamation, its Blueprint for mental health.[235] The Blueprint outlined $3.5B in proposed expenditure over five years on programs that were identified as mental health 'best buys'. The most expensive 'best buy' at $910 million was for establishing 20 new EPPICs.[236] The Blueprint stated that EPPIC had 'the largest international evidence base of any mental health model of care demonstrating not only their clinical effectiveness but also their financial and social return on investment'. Despite this bold claim, there was no evidence in the blueprint of EPPIC's cost effectiveness or patient outcomes compared with outcomes from other mental health services. To put it bluntly, this claim was bullshit.

The second most expensive program identified in the Blueprint was $226 million for the expansion of the national headspace program to 90 service sites. Other McGorry/Hickie pet projects also featured prominently, so the lion's share of funding was recommended to go to programs designed and controlled by them. The Blueprint was completely unreferenced. It was merely a consensus wish-list of these supposedly independent mental health experts led by McGorry, Hickie, and Cappo, that was devoid of supporting verifiable evidence. Neither did McGorry or Hickie or any other member of the Independent Reform Group disclose their pharmaceutical company connections in the Blueprint.

Minister Butler and the Gillard Government should have resisted the pressure applied by McGorry, Hickie, Cappo etc. and ordered an independent review of the evidence. They did not, and in May 2011, two months after the Blueprint was released, the Gillard Government announced $2.2 billion in funding for mental health. This included

$222.4 million (to be matched by state governments) to roll out '16 EPPIC sites nationally… [that] will have the capacity to assist more than 11,000 young Australians with, or at risk of developing, psychotic mental illness'.[237] [238]

Six months later, in September 2011, Monsignor Cappo was appointed by Prime Minister Gillard as the chair of the Mental Health Commission. However, within a week, he was asked to resigned because of allegations – that were already publicly known at the time of his appointment – that he did not act appropriately in relation to rape allegations against Catholic priests.[239] Monsignor Cappo was later cleared of any wrongdoing; however, his appointment and resignation within a week was emblematic of just how ham-fisted, ill-conceived and reactionary the Gillard Government's approach to the McGorry/Hickie driven demands for mental health were.

EPPIC/EPYS survive their first crisis

The May 2011 announcement by the American Psychiatric Association that Psychosis Risk Disorder (Attenuated Psychosis Syndrome) was not going to be recognised as a diagnosable disorder in DSM-5 was a significant obstacle for McGorry. EPPICs were being funded by taxpayers in part to diagnose and treat a psychiatric disorder that was not going to be officially recognised. The obvious question was: Why should Australian taxpayers fund the roll out of a new national early psychosis system based on a concept that has just been rejected internationally as unproven and dangerous?

When challenged on this, Professor McGorry responded by making the astonishing claim that 'EPPICs do not treat people with psychosis risk but only patients who have had their first psychotic episode'.[240] This was clearly contradictory to the Gillard Government's announcement and multiple previous and subsequent statements by Professor

McGorry. It also made no sense, given that the second P in EPPIC stands for Prevention.

In June 2011, Patrick McGorry's close colleague, Professor Alison Yung, also pushed the temporary McGorry party-line by claiming that EPPIC will not treat young people who are pre-psychotic.[241] Yung also claimed the debate about the pre-psychosis ultra-high risk syndrome is entirely separate from the role of EPPIC, which only treats people who already have psychosis. This was at odds with the EPPIC website, which stated that 'EPPIC also has a dedicated service for people thought to be at risk of developing a psychotic disorder, the PACE team.'[242] The Pace (Personal Assessment and Crisis Evaluation) offered a range of service options, including 'Specialised treatments, including psychological therapy and medication.'[243] Furthermore, the EPPIC clinical guidelines stated that siblings of EPPIC clients (and other people with an 'at risk' mental state) should be referred to PACE.[244] Clearly pre-emptive/preventive treatment was an important component of the EPPIC model, and potential patients were being actively recruited.

Perhaps at the time Hickie and Yung made these claims, treatment of those assessed as being at ultra-high risk of developing psychosis was planned to happen in another silo within the McGorry/EPPIC/headspace/PACE/Orygen youth mental health empire. So while they were possibly not lying, they were definitely not telling the whole – or even the most relevant part – of the truth.

There is no ambiguity that identifying those perceived to be at ultra-high risk was core to the McGorry early psychosis model in the minds of its potential funders. Like the Commonwealth Gillard Labor (Centre Left) Government, the Western Australian Barnett Liberal/National (Centre Right) Government – one of the six Australian state governments that it was hoped would match the Commonwealth Government's funding – believed this in May 2012, declaring that 'Early

Psychosis Prevention and Intervention Centre (EPPIC) services are for young people with first episode early psychosis and for detecting those with ultra-high risk of developing psychosis'.[245]

In response to the APA removing Psychosis Risk Disorder from the Draft of DSM-5, the Gillard Government should have pulled the funding immediately from the proposed EPPICs and redirected the funds to services with a sound evidence base and a proven record of helping young people. However, it seems Minister Butler and the Gillard Government – with the most fragile majority in Australian political history - lacked the appetite for a fight with a former Australian of the Year and media darling. McGorry's plans survived that obstacle, but hit a road block when individual state governments sensibly declined to kick in half the funding. Nonetheless, the Gillard Government agreed to solely fund some of the promised EPPICs.

Identifying those considered to be at ultra-high risk is still core business for McGorry-led early intervention services. As at October 2019, the Joondalup hYEPP (headspace Youth Early Psychosis Program) website stated that the service is available for:

> Young people [aged 12 to 25] who are experiencing their first episode of psychosis, or... who are at risk of developing psychosis. This may include young people who have a family history of psychosis, have a decline in functionality, and/or have transient psychotic symptoms.[246]

In addition, the national website for headspace states that headspace Early Psychosis Services are:

> ... in a unique position to identify and treat those at risk. Based on evidence developed by Orygen; the National Centre of Excellence in Youth Mental Health, the program focuses on early intervention, providing young people and their families with timely access to specialist support. headspace centres delivering

the early psychosis program are equipped with specially trained staff to help young people and their families.[247]

An example of the guidance offered by *Orygen* to the 'specially trained staff' is a *Comprehensive Assessment of At Risk Mental State (CAARMS) Training DVD*.[248] It trains staff on how to diagnose youth considered to be at ultra-high risk of becoming psychotic. Professor Yung (then an Associate Professor) introduces the video, stating:

> The CAARMS has two functions: First, to assess whether the person meets the ultra-high risk criteria for psychosis or not and second, to assess the range of psycho-pathology which we see typically in people in the prodrome preceding a first episode of psychosis. For this training video we'll just focus on the first function, that of assessing the ultra high-risk criteria… We're going to show you four interviews of typical people who present to the PACE clinic. Also in the DVD there will be slides showing the ratings for each of these people. By viewing the DVD you'll see both how the interviewer asks the questions and the responses that we commonly encounter at the clinic.

The interviewees in the training video were played by actors. The interviewer was a real clinician. An excerpt of the DVD showing a mock interview between a psychiatrist and an 18-year-old apprentice electrician Nick is available online.[249] In the excerpt, Nick explains how he feels pressured by his father to complete his apprenticeship and eventually take over the family business. Nick is anxious that he is not a good apprentice and it is obvious he feels bullied into following his father's plans for him.

At the end of the interview, Professor Yung explains why Nick meets the diagnostic criteria for being at ultra-high risk of psychosis (i.e. having Attenuated Psychosis Syndrome or Psychosis Risk Disorder).

In my non-clinical opinion, the evidence used to diagnose Nick is incredibly flimsy and demonstrates that the process is dangerously devoid of credibility.

Jon Jureidini, Professor of Psychiatry at Adelaide University, agrees with my assessment. In a commentary accompanying my video blog, he wrote that, rather than being a credible learning tool, the Orygen DVD 'provides a potential teaching tool for medical students in how not to carry out a psychiatric interview and interact with young people'.[250]

Professor Jureidini wrote:

> Nick is now being taught to see himself as sick. Who knows if this might not even increase this vulnerable young man's risk of ultimately being diagnosed with full-blown psychosis? And as Martin Whitely points out, it stigmatises him. But more important to me than stigmatisation is the fact that the UHR label is an unexplanation; it ignores what is going on in Nick's life. Unexplaining is different from saying 'I don't know' (something we doctors would do well to say more often). Unexplanations distract from the difficult but rewarding task of working with a young person towards finding an explanation for their stress.
>
> Nick makes it pretty easy for the listener. He tells us about being bullied into a trade that he does not want to be in, and he invites the interviewer to explore his relationship with his father. The interviewer does not notice, or chooses to ignore this invitation, instead sticking to a stereotyped list of questions that generate the sterile unexplanation of UHR. It might be argued that the interviewer would come back to this later. However, in my experience, young people prefer us to show an interest in their difficult and intimate predicaments when they first get the courage to put them into words.[251]

Another Australian psychiatrist, Dr Niall McLaren, wrote an unsolicited comment in September 2012 when the excerpt was published on a website I established.

> I have watched both segments of the Orygen training video and read the transcript. In my opinion, having had very long experience of people in this young man's position, any psychiatrist who diagnosed him as 'ultra-high risk of a psychotic disorder' is a dangerously incompetent psychiatrist. The diagnosis of an acute stress response in a vulnerable and exposed youth is crystal clear... Their decision to label this youth as 'pre-psychotic' was driven by their determination to diagnose this condition regardless of the reality factors, i.e. it was an ideological decision, not scientific.[252]

You don't need to be a psychiatrist to be concerned about how unscientific the process demonstrated in the DVD excerpt is. Watch the excerpt (available at https://www.psychwatchaustralia.com/mcgorry-video-fails-commonsense-tes), apply common sense, and decide for yourself: Is Nick sick with attenuated psychosis? Or is Nick simply very unhappy because he feels forced into a job he hates by his Dad and perhaps he smokes a bit too much dope?

Since this DVD was released in 2009, successive Australian Governments, of both the Centre Left and Centre Right, have committed hundreds of millions of taxpayer's dollars to a service built on this model. A model that diagnoses children as young as twelve as being pre-psychotic. I wonder if the Ministers and Prime Ministers responsible would have done this if they took the twenty minutes required to watch the excerpt of this DVD? I think not. It really is that bad!

I also doubt our political leaders considered the independent evidence regarding EPPICs. In June 2012, a systematic review assessing the cost of early intervention in psychosis conducted by Brisbane psychiatrist and economist Dr Andrew Amos was published in the *Australian and New Zealand Journal of Psychiatry*. The abstract states:

Results: Eleven articles were included in the review. The more rigorous research (two randomised control trials and two quasi-experimental studies) suggested no difference in resource utilisation or costs between early-intervention and treatment-as-usual groups. One small case-control study [co-authored by McGorry] with evidence of significant bias concluded annual early-intervention costs were one-third of treatment-as-usual costs. Conclusion: The published literature does not support the contention that early intervention for psychosis reduces costs or achieves cost-effectiveness. Past failed attempts to reduce health costs by reducing hospitalization, and increased outpatient costs in early-intervention programmes suggest such programmes may increase costs.[253]

Ultimately the lack of evidence didn't matter; McGorry's momentum was unstoppable. As McGorry had foretold in 2005, evidence was not 'an inhibitor or even prerequisite for exploration of reform'.[254]

EPPIC/EPYS survive their second crisis

Having survived the 2011-2012 crisis caused by the removal of Psychosis Risk Disorder from the draft of DSM-5 (that should have seen EPPICs defunded by the Gillard Government), EPPICs and McGorry faced a second crisis in June 2016. The Turnbull Coalition Government Health Minister Sussan Ley announced the staged closure of the seven Early Psychosis Services located at headspaces.

It was planned that the money saved would be redistributed to Primary Health Networks to spend on a broader range of youth focused services. In 2015, the Commonwealth Government established 31 Primary Health Networks in order to 'make sure government money is directed to where

it's needed and is spent on health programs that will be most effective'.
[255] Minister Ley told the ABC that the changes were part of a bank of
recommendations made by some of the country's top mental health
experts and the money would be allocated more effectively.[256]

Orygen Youth Health's (headed up by Patrick McGorry) website
describes how Professor McGorry went over Minister Ley's head and
publicly lobbied Prime Minister Turnbull to intervene at the eleventh
hour and save headspace Early Psychosis Services.[257]

Excerpt from
National Reform and the Roll-out of EPPIC[258]
18 October 2018

'By the end of 2014, most of the programs were being
implemented and were starting to do well. And then Sussan Ley
became Health Minister. That's when it really started to go pear-
shaped,' Professor McGorry says.

'At that point, a decision was made by senior bureaucrats and
supported by the Minister [Sussan Ley] to wind this program
up and hand over the funds to be used in a diffuse and "flexible"
manner by the new and untested Primary Health Networks on
completely non-evidence-based programs. Naturally, that caused
huge problems for the patients that were already being treated,
created serious risks and widespread distress, including for the
dedicated staff that were trying to make those programs work.

'It was a completely outrageous decision, which flew in the face of
arguably the best-quality evidence ever assembled for any model
of mental health care. We tried everything politically to get it
reversed in the lead-up to the 2016 election, but even with a fair
bit of support with the coalition, we couldn't get it reversed.'

In a last-ditch effort to save the programs, Professor McGorry addressed the National Press Club, accompanied by a young person from the program. The following Sunday, the *Sunday Telegraph* hit Sydney streets with the headline, 'Mal, Can We Talk? Funding cuts prompt fears of youth suicide rise', blazoned across the front. 'Within hours of that article being released, the Prime Minister was on the phone to me saying, "What do we need to do to fix this?" And within two hours, they organised a personal meeting with Sussan Ley, her adviser, Kerryn Pennell, myself – with Treasurer Scott Morrison and Malcolm Turnbull joining on the phone,' Professor McGorry remembers.

Elsewhere on this *National Reform and the Roll-out of EPPIC* webpage, Professor McGorry is described in heroic terms as having transformed from 'clinician-researcher to reform warrior' on a 'long and fraught… journey from inspiration and innovation to real-world implementation'. [259] The webpage cites no supporting evidence but includes a few personal stories of young people's lives supposedly transformed by EPPIC services.

In my experience, this is typical of McGorry's political approach. Addressing the media alongside young people his services have 'saved', and peddling fear of a spike in youth suicide if his services don't get more government funds, has proven very effective for McGorry. It is great salesmanship, but it is not science. Professor McGorry is brilliant at pulling at the heartstrings, and to date, it has almost always worked. He is frequently portrayed by the media as a humble, selfless, social justice warrior. In reality, he is a brilliant self-promoter and empire builder with extensive networks within government and industry.

Will EPPPIC/EPYS survive its third crisis?

At the time of writing this book, EPYS/EPPIC was facing a third threat to its Commonwealth Government funding. In the lead up to the May 2019 Australian Federal election, the Morrison Government had committed '$110 million to continue the Early Psychosis Youth Services [EPYS] program at six headspace centres nationally'.[260] The potential spanner in the works for ongoing EPYS funding is that the 2020 Productivity Commission's mental health report, commissioned by the Morrison Government, includes a bombshell recommendation, that would end headspace's and EPYS funding guarantee. Regional commissioning bodies that allocate Commonwealth Government to local services would be permitted "to redirect funding hypothecated to headspace centres and other particular providers to alternative services, subject to these services demonstrably not meeting the service needs identified in regional plans".[261]

This recommendation is potentially very bad news for McGorry. It threatens not only EPYS but also the monopoly that headspace has on Commonwealth Government funds for youth (aged 12 to 25 years) mental health services. The Productivity Commission basically recommended that the Government should step back and let Australia's 31 Primary Health Networks do their job, i.e. purchase, provide and integrate local health services. It is a very sensible recommendation, as there is very little independent, robust, evidence supporting the effectiveness of either headspace or EPYS.

It will be interesting to see how McGorry responds to this latest threat to both Early Psychosis Services and headspace. I wouldn't write off either program yet. McGorry is extraordinarily good at playing the game. It will require our politicians and the media to get beyond McGorry's former Australian of the Year status and scrutinise his Donald Trump-like boast that EPYS has 'the best-quality evidence ever'.

headspace – Does the hype match the reality?

Professor Patrick McGorry has frequently asserted that headspace is supported by extensive evidence. However, two external evaluations of headspace conducted in cooperation with headspace, and one independent assessment, do not support Professor McGorry's positive assertion.

The two evaluations conducted with headspace's cooperation both provided very weak evidence to support the effectiveness of headspace, let alone its cost-effectiveness. The first evaluation, Muir et al (2009), found 'there was little tangible evidence of the extent to which services were evidence-based'.[262] The more recent evaluation, Hilferty et al. (2015), showed high levels of client attrition and raised concerns about poor engagement with Indigenous young people.[263] Media reports have also raised similar concerns.[264]

Furthermore, even the weak evidence of positive outcomes in these two reviews is questionable, because both evaluations had significant methodological limitations. The Muir 2009 evaluation had no control group for comparison.[265] Hilferty et al.'s 2015 evaluation used two comparison groups.[266] The 18-25-year-old comparison group was recruited online from commercial access panels, with a very low response rate (p. 175), and was poorly-matched (p. 16). In addition, the headspace client survey group excluded clients who only attended once (p. 180), and girls/women were over-represented (p. 179).

The independent assessment conducted in 2015 by Professor Anthony Jorm, without headspace's involvement, found 'improvements seen in headspace clients are similar to those seen in untreated cases, and it would seem that the services provided may have had little or no effect'.[267] Apart from the weak evidence base, other concerns associated with the rollout of headspace include problems with workforce shortages and its failure to service those most at risk and respond to local conditions.

In September 2019, headspace was described by three psychiatrists in the *Australian New Zealand Journal of Psychiatry* as a Leviathan swallowing resources in a haphazard uncoordinated manner.[268] In 2014, the National Mental Health Commission (NHMC) concluded that headspace was:

> an example of the Commonwealth entering into areas of direct service provision which were previously the domain of the states and territories. Although headspace has been a "game changer" in terms of adolescent mental health, the need for each headspace centre to integrate and coordinate with state services has been under emphasised and under achieved.[269]

The NHMC also concluded that headspace centres were set up without adequate consultation resulting in the 'duplication of, and competition with, other community, private and state government services'.[270]

All of these considerations aside, a huge part of the rationale for establishing headspace centres was to reduce rates of youth suicide. In this regard, as demonstrated in Chapter 2, headspace has been an abject failure.

As *Time* magazine had identified in 2006, for McGorry, contradictory evidence doesn't inhibit his 'full steam ahead, damn the torpedoes' enthusiasm.[271] McGorry went close to acknowledging his propensity to push forward despite the evidence in a paper published in the *British Journal of Psychiatry* in 2005 that stated:

> In psychiatric as well as other reform processes, logic and scientific evidence are necessary but insufficient. Rhetoric, marketing, effective networking, altruistic promotion of a vital public health issue, economic arguments and a confluence of common interests have fuelled the momentum and are vital for real reform to take root... We do need evidence as a tool and guide and ally but not as an inhibitor or even prerequisite for exploration of reform. Evidence is the language of reform but

there are other language of reform but there are other elements in communication. There is also rhetoric, prosody [rhythmic poetic language] persuasion and at the heart of things, a chorus of voices reflecting the human experience of illness and recovery. The latter can be a uniquely powerful force for change. We sense that a large rock has been cast into the lake of psychiatry. The ripples are spreading. In time they may spread to all shores to help to improve the survival and quality of life for all people affected by psychotic disorders. In turn, the prospects for psychiatry as a whole and all those bearing the hidden burden of mental disorders may correspondingly improve.272

Professor McGorry is unquestionably an exceptionally effective marketer, networker and lobbyist. He has used 'rhetoric, prosody' and orchestrated a 'chorus of voices' to persuade most of the media, and all of the key politicians, that he can 'improve the survival and quality of life for all people affected by psychotic disorders'. And he has done all this without letting a lack of robust supporting evidence act 'as an inhibitor or even prerequisite for exploration of reform'.[273]

Disease-Mongering

Along with claiming that the programs he developed are 'shovel-ready'[274] to deliver proven 21st century solutions, McGorry also repeatedly sells the message that there is massive unmet need. In March 2010 when appearing on ABC TV's Lateline program, McGorry said:

Four million Australians have mental health problems in any given year. Only one third of them get access to treatment... there are one million young Australians aged 12 to 25 with a mental disorder in any given year. It's the peak period across a lifespan when mental disorders appear. And 750,000 of them have no access to mental health care currently.[275 276]

Public critics were rare; however, not everyone accepted McGorry's alarming claims. Adelaide University Professor of Psychiatry and Paediatrics, and Head of the Department of Psychological Medicine at the Women's and Children's Hospital in Adelaide, Jon Jureidini, accused McGorry of disease-mongering when claiming that 750,000 young Australians were denied care:

> He's taken the biggest possible figure you can come up with for people who might have any level of distress or unhappiness, which of course needs to be taken seriously and responded to, but he's assuming they all require... a mental health intervention... It's the way politicians operate. You look at figures and put a spin on it that suits your point of view. I don't think that has a place in scientific conversations about the need for health interventions.[277]

McGorry responded to Jureidini's criticisms writing, 'I have never argued that one million young Australians have serious mental illness'.[278] But he then immediately contradicted himself by stressing how serious mild to moderate mental illness is:

> To argue that young Australians with mild to moderate mental ill-health do not need access to mental health care applies a standard to mental health that would not be acceptable in physical health. Imagine restricting access to health services to only Australians with severe physical ill-health and locking out all those with milder conditions with the admonition that they should just regard their distress as part of the human condition and suck it up![279]

However, it is not true that these young Australians are all locked out of services they desperately need. Many adolescents and young adults that McGorry would regard as experiencing 'mild to moderate mental ill-health' don't seek help, often because they don't want it.

Many young people are resilient and consider their current depressed mood or anxiety is not a product of their underlying mental illness, but rather a product of their personal circumstances. Many do just choose to 'suck it up' and understand that sometimes 'shit happens'. They don't catastrophise adversity and medicalise their misery in the way that McGorry and others promote.

Equating mental illness with physical illness is a common debating tactic of McGorry when arguing for greater resources for his mental health programs. Despite often being treated with a medicalised response in hospitals, or doctor surgeries, in reality mental illness and physical illness have little else in common. Many physical illnesses, such as cancer, type 1 diabetes and haemochromatosis, have physical or genetic biomarkers from blood test, scans, or a host of other objective diagnostic tests. Mental Illness does not. Physical illnesses can often be cured by short duration drug treatment, whereas the drugs used to treat mental illness at best temporarily manage symptoms, but never cure the condition. It is a neat debating trick to equate the two but it does not stand scrutiny.

Professor McGorry also characterised Professor Jureidini as a proponent of 'the late intervention philosophy' which he argued:

> is associated with risk, preventable damage and stigma and for this reason access to appropriate, staged mental health care for young Australians with mild, moderate and serious mental ill-health is overwhelmingly supported by political parties and the health and social sectors (most recently expressed in a letter co-signed by 65 organisations).[280]

Again, it is a neat debating trick to characterise his critics as proponents of late intervention; but opposing pre-emptive intervention, particularly labelling and drugging before diagnosis, is not a late-intervention approach. Nonetheless, McGorry was correct in identifying that there appeared to be 'overwhelming' support 'by political parties' for his approach. However, this is evidence of political rather than clinical or scientific success. Arguably McGorry's elevation to Australian of the Year in an election year almost guaranteed him bipartisan support. After all, what aspiring political leader about to face the voters is going to pick a fight with an officially endorsed national hero (i.e. Australian of the Year) about their area of expertise?

McGorry is on stronger ground with his claim that 'Four million Australians have mental health problems in any given year'. As mentioned in Chapter 1, according to reputable sources, including the Australian Bureau of Statistics, well over four million Australians are suffering from a mental illness. In fact, the most recent Australian Bureau of Statistics National Health Survey estimated there were 4.8 million Australians (20.1% of the population) with a mental or behavioural condition in 2017–18.281 This was an increase of 2.6 percentage points from 2014–15, mainly due to an increase in the number of people reporting anxiety-related conditions, depression, or feelings of depression.

The problem is that these four million-plus estimates are based on DSM-5 diagnostic criteria. Given how wide DSM-5 casts the mental illness net, it is surprising the number isn't even higher. By narrowing the boundaries of normality, massive numbers can be classified as mentally ill.

In addition, as discussed in Chapter 1, there are methodological flaws in surveys designed to determine the prevalence of mental illness. These flaws almost always result in survey participants who are temporarily distressed but would never buy into the DSM-5 framework by being identified as having a psychiatric disorder. All this results in massive estimates of the prevalence of mental illness and unmet need. This suits the purposes of mental health entrepreneurs like McGorry.

The short attention span of Australian policy makers and media has also benefitted McGorry. As discussed above, he has spun his position on a number of issues, but has rarely been held to account. Changing your position in the face of emerging evidence or because you have been convinced by alternative arguments is commendable. However, spinning your position in order to overcome temporary obstacles posed by contradictory evidence, or a change in public sentiment, should not be acceptable from a scientist advising on important aspects of public policy. If the science supporting McGorry's original positions – particularly his support for the formal recognition of psychosis risk disorder – was as robust as he previously claimed, there would have been no need for so many significant flip-flops.

Chapter 6

ADHD: So Big It Must Be Real?

ADHD is big business – very big business. In 2018, global sales of ADHD drugs totalled US$16.4 billion (approximately A$25 billion) and are forecast to rise to US$25 billion by 2025.[282] This does not include the tens of billions earned by those who diagnose, research and otherwise make a living from ADHD. The massive industry is built on the increasingly discredited theory that ADHD is caused by a biochemical brain dysfunction. The highly dubious assumption being that the medications, primarily amphetamines, correct the imbalance and allow the ADHD sufferer to function normally. In effect, ADHD is treated as if it is caused by a deficit of amphetamine.

Despite 30 years of hyped but unfulfilled promises of imminent technological diagnostic breakthroughs, there are no brain scans, blood tests or other objective physical tests for ADHD. DSM-5 states that 'no biological marker is diagnostic for ADHD',[283] and it details the behavioural diagnostic criteria that are the sole basis for a diagnosis (listed below). Every claim about ADHD should be viewed in light of these criteria.

Extract from the
**Diagnostic and Statistical Manual of Mental Disorders 5th Edition
DSM-5 ADHD Diagnostic Criteria[284]**

To meet the DSM-5 diagnostic criteria a child should display either:

- six of the behavioural criteria below at 1 (Predominantly Inattentive Subtype – sometimes referred to as passive ADHD or ADD)

- six of the behavioural criteria below at 2 (Predominantly Hyperactive/Impulsive Subtype)

- or six of both 1 and 2 (Combined Subtype)

for at least six months to an extent that is inconsistent with their age and significantly impairs their social and academic functioning. For adolescents 17+ and adults five are sufficient.

1. Inattention

- often fails to give close attention to details or **makes careless mistakes** in schoolwork, work, or during other activities

- often has **difficulty sustaining attention** in tasks or play activities

- often **does not seem to listen** when spoken to directly

- often does not follow through on instructions and **fails to finish schoolwork, chores,** or duties in the workplace

- often has **difficulty organizing tasks** and activities

- often **avoids, dislikes** or is reluctant to engage in tasks that require sustained mental effort (such as schoolwork or **homework**)

- often **loses things** necessary for tasks or activities (e.g., toys, school assignments, pencils, books, or tools)

- is often **easily distracted** by extraneous stimuli

- is **often forgetful** in daily activities

2. Hyperactivity and Impulsivity

- often **fidgets** with hands or feet or squirms in seat

- often **leaves seat** in classroom or in other situations in which remaining seated is expected

- often **runs about or climbs excessively** in situations in which it is inappropriate

- often **unable to play** or engage in leisure activities **quietly**

- is often **'on the go'** or often acts as if 'driven by a motor'

- often **talks excessively**

- often **blurts out answers** before questions have been completed

- often **has difficulty awaiting turn**

- often **interrupts or intrudes** on others (e.g., butts into conversations or games)

DSM-5 also recognises two additional categories of ADHD where children 'do not meet the full criteria for ADHD'.

- Other Specified ADHD – when clinician 'chooses to communicate the specific reason that the presentation does not meet the criteria for ADHD'.

- Unspecified ADHD – when the clinician 'chooses not to communicate the specific reason that the presentation does not meet' these criteria.

In my experience, when ordinary Australians are shown the diagnostic criteria for ADHD, they respond in one of two ways. The most common response is 'WTF? That is bullshit… fidgeting, disliking homework, playing loudly etc. are all normal childhood behaviours'.

The minority response is 'Oh my god that is my child and/or that's me... My child and/or I must have ADHD'.

However, most people never see these criteria and simply assume there must be solid science underpinning the diagnosis. Like the Emperor's New Clothes, they believe ADHD must be a legitimate illness, because so many other seemingly credible people, including highly credentialed medical professionals, claim to be able to see it. In simple terms, they conclude ADHD is so big that it must be real.

Many of the criticisms of the disorder (lack of objective diagnostic tests, diagnostic creep, overselling of the benefits of medications) apply to other psychiatric disorders. It is the medicalisation of normal (if annoying) childhood behaviours that sets ADHD apart. The symptoms of severe depression, schizophrenia and bipolar disorder are extreme behaviours, but even many ADHD proponents acknowledge there is nothing unusual about children fidgeting, running, playing loudly and disliking homework.

What is supposed to distinguish ADHD sufferers from the rest of the population is that they exhibit these behaviours so 'often' that they significantly interfere with the child's functioning. Specifically, 'There must be clear evidence that the symptoms interfere with, or reduce the quality of, social, academic or occupational functioning' and 'Several inattentive or hyperactive –impulsive symptoms are present in two or more settings (e.g. at home, school; with friends or relatives; in other activities)'.[285] How 'often' a child 'fidgets or squirms in their seat', or 'interrupts' or 'avoids homework' or 'fails to remain seated when remaining seated is expected' or 'is distracted by external stimuli' so that they 'interfere' with the child's 'functioning' is not defined in DSM-5. Like beauty, 'impairment' is in the eye of the beholder.

DSM-IV also says:

Signs of the disorder may be minimal or absent when the

individual is receiving frequent rewards for appropriate behaviour, is under close supervision, is in a novel setting, is engaged in especially interesting activities, has consistent external stimulation (e.g., via electronic screens), or is interacting in a one-to-one situation (e.g., the clinician's office.)[286]

In other words, ADHD children will behave appropriately and not display symptoms when they are rewarded, when people pay attention to them (close supervision) and when they are having new experiences. Conversely, ADHD children will be inattentive, easily distracted and display ADHD symptoms when their good behaviour goes unrewarded, no one pays any attention to them, or they are bored.

The biggest market for ADHD drugs is boys. All across the globe, boys are roughly three to four times more likely than girls to be medicated. It is not hard to understand why. There are many exceptions, but boys are generally wired to be risk takers, louder, more impulsive, less mature, more competitive and less cooperative than girls. The plain truth is that, on average, boys are more annoying, and display more challenging behaviours than girls. Given that we drug ADHD children because their behaviour is a problem, it makes perfect sense that we drug way more boys than girls.

The ADHD Industry has recognised that girls are an under-exploited market. In response, they have made a significant effort to market 'passive ADHD' (or ADD without the H for hyperactivity) as a gender equity issue. The argument is that 'quiet daydreaming girls' are believed to be missing out as their 'disability' is being 'under-recognised'. There is some evidence that the gender gap is slowly closing, but only because the prescribing rates for girls maybe rising even faster than that for boys. One of the disturbing drivers of this trend may be the use, particularly by teenage girls and young women, of stimulants to get thin.[287]

The other great marketing push in recent years has been in selling 'adult ADHD'. It has been very successful, with the numbers of Australian adults prescribed ADHD medications jumping from 37,134 in 2013 to 57,605 in 2017.[288] This is not surprising. Selling amphetamine to adults has never been difficult. Taken in moderate doses, amphetamines make most people feel alert, focussed and on top of their game. Convincing some adults that they can only be their best self with amphetamines in their system is easy and profitable.

DSM-5 was a great leap forward in marketing ADHD. The final version of DSM-5, published in May 2013, made it significantly easier to qualify for a diagnosis of ADHD, but it could have been even easier. An early draft of DSM-5, released for public comment, proposed the inclusion of four extra ways of exhibiting impulsivity:

1. Tends to act without thinking.
2. Is often impatient.
3. Is uncomfortable doing things slowly and systematically.
4. Finds it difficult to resist temptations or opportunities.

This early draft also proposed that, for anyone aged 17 or older, the ADHD diagnostic threshold was proposed to be lowered further. If the proposed changes were adopted, it would be sufficient to meet as few as four (down from six) of either the nine inattentive or four of the proposed expanded 13 impulsive/hyperactive criteria.[289] Following a considerable backlash, the final version of DSM-5 was tightened a little from what was proposed in the draft. Most notably the four extra criteria were not included.

Nonetheless, the changes between DSM-IV and DSM-5 were significant, with an emphasis on making it easier to diagnose ADHD in adults. For those aged 17 or over, the number of criteria that had to be displayed was reduced from six to five. The final DSM-5 also relaxed the DSM-IV requirement that signs of the behaviour should be displayed before age seven. It is now sufficient to display some symptoms before age twelve. Other significant loosening of the criteria from DSM-IV to DSM-5 included:

1. The relaxation of the expectation that teachers independently provide evidence.[290]
2. Replacing hyperactive actions in the wording of criteria to feelings or perceptions of 'restlessness'.
3. Pathologising the normal phenomena that ADHD behaviours are 'typically more marked during times when the person is studying or working' than 'during vacation'.
4. The inclusion of adult relevant examples in most of the diagnostic criteria which had previously been primarily orientated to children in a school setting.[291]

All of these changes made the already extraordinarily loose DSM-IV criteria even looser and encouraged increased diagnosis and treatment. The criteria fall way short of what constitutes a valid, science based, psychiatric diagnosis. The idea that reports of children behaving like children – playing, climbing, running, talking, not waiting their turn, interrupting, and avoiding homework etc. – is evidence of a psychiatric disorder is just absurd. It is even more absurd that the first line treatment for this 'disorder' is to give children – sometimes even toddlers – a daily amphetamine habit. But this is precisely what we do to vast numbers of Australian children.

130,000+ Aussie kids take drugs for ADHD in 2019

In 2009, according to the Australian Government data, 60,931 children were dispensed at least one prescription of an ADHD medication (primarily amphetamines).[292] In 2017, the latest year for which age specific data is available, this number had risen to 107,345.[293] Since then (from January 2018 until September 2019), the total number of Australian PBS subsidised prescriptions has risen at 11% per annum.[294]

Based on this rate of growth, I estimate that more than 130,000 Australian children were dispensed an ADHD medication in 2019. In summary, from 2009 until 2019, the percentage of Australian children aged 4-17 years dispensed ADHD drugs has grown from 1.6% to an estimated 3.0%.

The vast majority of drugs prescribed to treat ADHD are psychostimulants containing dexamphetamine (brand names Adderall, Dexedrine, Dexostrat, Vyvanse) and the near amphetamine methylphenidate (Ritalin, Concerta, Attenta).[295] Other non-stimulant drugs less commonly used include Atomoxetine Hydrochloride (brand name Strattera) and occasionally Clonidine (brand name Kapvay)[296] and Guanfacine (brand name Intuniv)[297]. All carry significant warnings for potential adverse effects. Although not available in Australia, methamphetamine (brand name Desoxyn[298]), is available in the USA to treat children as young as six. All ADHD drugs have significant potential adverse effects.[299] They range from common short-term effects like insomnia, loss of appetite and headaches, through to severe cardiovascular and psychiatric problems, addiction, growth retardation and suicide.

The massive explosion in prescribing rates in Australia, and across the globe, is evidence of the incredible marketing skills of the ADHD Industry. This marketing triumph has been so successful that my view – i.e. annoying, disruptive childhood behaviours are not evidence of a disease, and that amphetamines are bad for developing brains and bodies – is now a radical position.

A very common claim made by the ADHD Industry is that prevalence rates exceed diagnosis and treatment rates so, rather than being over-diagnosed and over-medicated, ADHD is massively under-diagnosed and under-treated. For diseases like asthma, haemochromatosis, or leukaemia – with science-based diagnosis, real and indisputable negative consequences, and medically valid treatments – we need to be concerned if prevalence rates exceed diagnosis rates. This means that real treatable disease is going undiagnosed. However, for subjective, ill-defined diagnosis like ADHD estimating the prevalence rate is like answering the question: How long is a piece of string? The answer depends entirely on how you cut it.

Estimates of the prevalence of ADHD have varied between 1.7%[300] and 29%[301] of children. This huge range is an inevitable consequence of relying on second hand reports of children fidgeting, interrupting, losing things etc. to diagnose a hypothetical neurodevelopmental psychiatric disorder.

It is important to understand that arguing that ADHD is a fraud, is different from claiming that all children diagnosed with ADHD are well. Some clearly do have problems and need support that matches their individual circumstances. Many non-biological factors have been associated with higher rates of ADHD diagnosis and medication use. These include gender, ethnicity of students and teachers[302], divorce[303], poverty[304], parenting styles[305], low maternal education, lone parenthood and the receipt of social welfare[306], sexual abuse[307], sleep deprivation[308], perinatal issues[309], artificial food additives[310], mobile phone use[311], clinician speciality[312], postcode and regulatory capture[313]. Children with behavioural problems need to have the causes of their individual circumstances identified and responded to. They do not need a daily amphetamine habit.

The attraction of amphetamines is that, while responses vary between individuals, there is no doubt that in most cases low dose psychostimulants narrow focus, and make disruptive children more compliant and easier to manage. This occurs in most people regardless of whether they are diagnosed with ADHD or not.[314]

These immediate behavioural changes are often welcomed by parents, teachers, and in some cases other students who benefit from not having to put up with annoying behaviour. The losers in this process are the 'medicated children', especially those with real problems that, because they are covered over with drugs, are never identified and addressed. Too often ADHD drugs mask the signs of serious problems such as sexual, emotional or physical abuse, bullying or trauma. Some children are doubly abused when the original abuse is compounded by the harmful administration of amphetamines. It's obvious that children who have been sexually or physically abused are highly likely to be inattentive and behave inappropriately. These blameless, voiceless, victims deserve the very best of care. Instead children who have been bashed or raped are told their brain is broken and they get a daily drug habit.

I recall a phone call when I was a member of the Western Australian Parliament from a grandmother whose nine-year-old granddaughter had been a victim of sustained sexual abuse by a family member. She was distraught that her daughter had allowed the young girl to be 'medicated' for ADHD. On dexamphetamine her granddaughter had become quiet and withdrawn, which apparently pleased her mother, but exasperated the grandmother who believed her real issues were being ignored.

The mother's response was common. When they see a quiet compliant 'medicated' child, in the minds of many parents, this is evidence that their child's 'biochemical imbalance' has been balanced. When the drugs wear off, however, there are often 'bounce' or withdrawal effects that worsen ADHD-type behaviours. Indeed, 'rebound' or withdrawal effects can occur that are 'often worse than the child's original or baseline behaviour', even after a single dose.[315]

The ADHD Industry has long known there is nothing ADHD specific about psychostimulants. In 1996 Dr Debra Zarin, representing the American Psychiatric Association and the American Academy of Child and Adolescent Psychiatry, testified to a US Congressional committee that:

It is a commonly held misconception that if a stimulant calms a child, that he must have ADHD; if he didn't have the disorder, the thinking goes, the medication would not have any effect. That is not true. Stimulants increase attention span in normal children as well as those with ADHD.[316]

Nonetheless, many within the industry aggressively promote the claim that if a low dose stimulant narrows focus or calms a child then they must have ADHD. This deceit has extended to the use of stimulants as a diagnostic tool.[317] The fallacious logic given is that if an ADHD diagnosed child's behaviour changes after taking stimulants, this confirms the diagnosis.

Another common myth about psychostimulants used to treat ADHD is that they are 'smart drugs'. In low doses they can allow an individual to concentrate on an assigned task, however, they inhibit creativity[318] and there is evidence that long-term exposure to stimulants to treat ADHD may cause dopamine system malfunctions (i.e. brain damage) that never existed before.[319] Diverted psychostimulants are frequently used by students to stay awake, focus longer and forgo sleep in an attempt to increase available study time in the lead up to exams. There is very little evidence that this actually helps.[320] US research found the misuse of these medications by college students for study purposes 'appears to be *negatively* associated with academic performance, indicating that misuse may not necessarily lead to academic enhancement, despite students' perceptions of their benefits'.[321] Some students report increased output in written exams but have expressed concerns they have swapped quality for quantity.[322]

Regardless of the short-term effects, real world data from Canada and Western Australia indicates that rather than being 'smart drugs', in the long-term their use is associated with declining academic performance. The Canadian study, published in 2014, followed the long term educational outcomes of 8,643 children in Quebec of whom 9% had ever used stimulants for ADHD by age 16.[323] The academic performance of the children medicated with stimulants for ADHD relative to their peers declined significantly in the years after commencing medication. The Quebec study also found ADHD medicated children experienced deteriorations in 'relationships with [their] parents' and 'increases in the probability that a child has ever suffered from depression'.[324] The much smaller, and therefore less definitive Western Australian study, concluded that among ADHD diagnosed children 'ever receiving stimulant medication was found to increase the odds of being identified as performing below age level by a classroom teacher by a factor of 10.5 times'. [325]

A significant part of the rationale for 'medicating' ADHD diagnosed children is the hypothesis that managing the symptoms of ADHD with stimulants 'allows children to learn skills and concepts' and that this helps children to achieve improved long term academic outcomes. [326] The long-term data from the natural experiments in Quebec Canada and to a lesser extent Western Australia provide disturbing evidence that the use of stimulants to treat ADHD may significantly impede long-term academic outcomes.

There has been a paucity of research into the long-term effects of ADHD medications. This may well be a case of wilful ignorance, where the ADHD Industry deliberately avoid finding out the truth about the lasting impact of their drugs on children.

One of the few well-resourced and sustained investigations into the long-term outcomes was the *Multimodal Treatment Study for Attention Deficit Hyperactivity Disorder* (the MTA Study). Up until 2007 it was probably the most cited source justifying the use of amphetamine type stimulants for ADHD. While there were several methodological flaws, notably a lack of a placebo and blind raters[327], the MTA Study did follow a significant number of children.[328] In 1999 after conducting the first fourteen months of the study the authors concluded that 'carefully crafted medication management was superior to the behavioural treatment and to routine clinical care that included medication'.[329] It was described as 'one of the first studies to demonstrate benefits of multimodal and pharmacological interventions lasting longer than 1 year' and became, I believe, the most frequently quoted single source supporting the use of stimulants for ADHD.[330]

However, in 2007, after an analysis of the three-year follow-up to the MTA Study, one of the scientists who ran the study, Professor William Pelham, concluded:

> I think we exaggerated the beneficial impact of medication in the first study. We had thought that children medicated longer would have better out-comes. That didn't happen to be the case... In the short run [medication] will help the child behave better, in the long run it won't. And that information should be made very clear to parents.[331]

The three-year data also showed that children using behavioural therapy alone had 'a slightly lower rate of substance abuse' and that 'the (medicated) children had a substantial decrease in their rate of growth, so they weren't growing as much as other kids in terms of both their height and their weight'.[332] [333] A further follow up study after 16 years demonstrated that the 'extended use of medication was associated with suppression of adult height but not with reduction of [ADHD] symptom severity'.[334]

The fact that the fourteen-month data supported the use of stimulants and the three-year and sixteen-year data did not, is also entirely in keeping with the commonsense proposition that children mature at different rates and 'that brains of children [diagnosed] with ADHD, rather than developing abnormally (as in autism), mature later'.[335] It also supports the idea that while nothing affects behaviour as fast as behaviour-altering medications, amphetamines simply mask symptoms and do nothing to address their cause.

The clearest evidence of how irredeemably flawed the ADHD label is (and how poorly modern schools cope with immaturity), comes from research I led with seven international co-authors. We used data for over 15 million children in 13 countries that demonstrated that across the globe the youngest children in a classroom are much more likely than their oldest classmates (up to a year older) to be 'medicated' for ADHD.[336] In effect, perfectly normal age-related immaturity among relatively young children is being treated as if it is a brain disorder.

This ADHD late birthdate effect occurs in countries with both high prescribing rates, like the USA and Canada, and low prescribing rates like Finland and Sweden. Our global research built on the earlier research I led that showed the youngest children in Western Australian primary school classrooms (born in June) are about twice as likely to be given ADHD drugs as their oldest classmates born the previous July.[337] Not surprisingly, in our Western Australian study and in most of the international studies we later examined, the effect was stronger in the early years of school, when as a proportion of time lived, the age difference between the youngest and oldest in class was greatest. Since our global study was first published in October 2018 multiple other studies have found the same effect.[338] [339]

Prior to the publication of our global analysis Professor Allen Frances, cited studies from the USA[340], Canada[341], and Iceland[342], as providing conclusive proof ADHD is over-diagnosed.[343] Professor Frances has repeatedly been critical of US prescribing rates and has argued that a diagnostic rate of around 2% to 3% would best balance harms and benefits.[344] However, the data from the large Swedish[345], Finnish[346], Taiwanese[347] and Western Australian[348] studies, and a much smaller Spanish[349] study, all showed strong late birthdate effects at rates of prescribing below Frances' estimated ideal target range. The fact that this happens in both high and low prescribing jurisdictions does not support Professor Frances' assertion that there is an ideal target range. Instead this indicates that misdiagnosis is an inevitable consequence of ADHD's extremely vague and broad diagnostic criteria, and that there is no safe level of diagnosis and prescribing.

As detailed in prior chapters Professor Frances deserves tremendous credit for his leading role in combatting Big Pharma's disease-mongering including the massive explosion in ADHD prescribing rates. However, it seems that recognising that this evidence shows that as a diagnostic entity ADHD is so fundamentally flawed that it must be abandoned, is a step too far for Professor Frances.[350]

When the journal articles demonstrating the ADHD late birthday effect have been published, they have generated considerable media coverage. The West Australian study won the award for having the largest media coverage of any research conducted at Curtin University in 2017.[351] The global study attracted even more interest, achieving the highest Altmetric Attention score of any article ever published in the prominent *Journal of Child Psychiatry and Psychology*.[352] However, this media coverage lasts a day, maybe two if you are lucky, whereas the ADHD Industry marketing machine rolls on 365 days a year. The efforts of unpaid ADHD critics, like me, can never beat the massive resources and professionalism of the ADHD Industry.

The response of the ADHD Industry to the late birthdate effect was to do what it usually does in response to inconvenient truths; it substantially ignored it. There were a few isolated comments from ADHD experts praising the research as demonstrating a real effect but suggesting that the problem wasn't that the youngest in class were over-diagnosed, rather the oldest in class with ADHD were being missed and not receiving the treatment they desperately need.

At least these few 'experts' deserve credit for engaging with the evidence, for many ADHD True Believers contradictory evidence simply doesn't matter. They have faith that ADHD is biological in origin and nothing can shake them from this belief. Many share an almost evangelical zeal about ADHD awareness raising. Their response to criticism of the 'science' of ADHD is anything but scientific, and is often highly emotional, as if you are attacking an unquestionable truth.

One example was the response by Sydney paediatrician and prominent ADHD expert Associate Professor Michael Kohn to an article in the *Daily Telegraph* highlighting adverse events reported to the TGA of psychosis and suicide attempts by children taking Ritalin.[353] Dr Kohn responded, 'This is the latest in a series of articles blaspheming the use of Ritalin in the treatment of behavioural disturbance in children.'[354]

Prominent ADHD 'experts' like Dr Kohn are often venerated by true believers, for their special insight that enable them to detect the disorder. A notable example is the US ADHD support group CHADD honouring high-profile ADHD ideologues in its 'ADHD Hall of Fame'. Inductees include Distinguished Professor of Psychiatry at the University of Utah School of Medicine, Paul Wender.[355] In 1995 Wender claimed to have found the holy grail of the ADHD movement, a reliable biological marker, *foot tapping*! According to Wender:

> Fidgeting and foot movements (known in our research setting as 'Wender's sign') are very common signs of hyperactivity in adult ADHD patients – so much so that such patients can usually be diagnosed in the waiting room by a knowledgeable receptionist... I seriously entertain the possibility that this foot movement may be a biological marker for ADHD[356]... [T]he reduction of the foot sign in ADHD patients may also be an indicator of stimulant [drug] response.[357]

That Wender was held in high enough regard by CHADD to be

inducted into the *ADHD Hall of Fame* speaks volumes about the credibility of both.

Wender's wild theory may be extreme, but it is typical of the ADHD Industry's substitution of speculation for science. If asked for proof of the medications' effectiveness, 'experts' will often respond that there are thousands of scientific papers that support their claims. When asked which one of these scientific papers has robust methodology, they cannot identify a single long-term research paper that withstands scrutiny.

Compelling evidence for the poor quality of this research was demonstrated in 2005 through the *Oregon Health and Science University ADHD Drug Effectiveness Review* Project. The review was commissioned by fifteen US states in order to determine which drugs were the safest and most cost effective.[358] The 731-page review analysed 2287 studies, 'virtually every investigation ever done on ADHD drugs anywhere in the world'.[359] Of the studies analysed, 'The group rejected 2,107 investigations as being unreliable, and reviewed the remaining 180 to find superior drugs'.[360] Instead of being able to make objective comparisons of the safety and effectiveness of the different drugs, the review was 'severely limited' by a lack of studies measuring 'functional or long-term outcomes'.[361]

The review concluded that 'evidence on the effectiveness of pharmacotherapy for ADHD in young children is seriously lacking'[362] and that there was 'no evidence on long-term safety of drugs used to treat ADHD in adolescents'[363]. The review also found that 'good quality evidence on the use of drugs to affect outcomes relating to global academic performance, consequences of risky behaviours, social achievements, etc. is lacking'.[364] It was also critical of the lack of research into the possibility that some ADHD drugs could stunt growth and found that the evidence that ADHD drugs help adults was 'not compelling'.[365] Overall, the review ascertained that the body of evidence was of 'poor quality'. Predictably these findings were either ignored or dismissed with the ADHD Industry mantra that the benefits of drugs 'clearly outweigh the risks'.[366]

Little has changed in the fifteen years since the *Oregon Health and Science University ADHD Drug Effectiveness Review* was published. Despite this paucity of evidence on the long-term effects of psycho-stimulants on children, parents are commonly reassured that stimulants have been used to control ADHD-like behaviour since the 1930s. This begs the obvious question: why haven't the pharmaceutical companies set up credible long-term analysis of the effects of their products? The answer is even more obvious: Why kill the goose that lays the golden eggs?

Consensus substituted for Science

ADHD experts don't draw their credibility from science. They can't. They simply don't have solid evidence to support the tenets of their faith. They draw their credibility from agreeing with other self-appointed ADHD experts. Consensus rather than science has driven the expansion of the definition of ADHD and changes in its diagnosis and treatment.

In 2002, a self-declared 'independent consortium' of eighty-four 'leading scientists' signed the 'International Consensus Statement on ADHD'. The first signatory was the world's most high-profile ADHD advocate, American psychologist Dr Russell Barkley who has been a paid speaker and consultant for most of the ADHD drug manufacturers including Eli Lilly, McNeil, Janssen-Orth, Janssen-Cilag, Novartis, Shire, and Theravance.[367]

Extract from the 'International Consensus Statement on ADHD'

This is the first consensus statement issued by an independent consortium of leading scientists concerning the status of the disorder. Among scientists who have devoted years, if not entire careers, to the study of this disorder there is no controversy regarding its existence... We cannot over emphasize the point that, as a matter of science, the notion that ADHD does not exist is simply wrong... the occasional coverage of the disorder casts the story in the form of a sporting event with evenly matched competitors. The views of a handful of non-expert doctors that ADHD does not exist are contrasted against mainstream scientific views that it does, as if both views had equal merit. Such attempts at balance give the public the impression that there is substantial scientific disagreement over whether ADHD is a real medical condition. In fact, there is no such disagreement – at least no more so than there is over whether smoking causes cancer, for example, or whether a virus causes HIV/AIDS... To publish stories that ADHD is a fictitious disorder or merely a conflict between today's Huckleberry Finns and their caregivers is tantamount to declaring the earth flat, the laws of gravity debatable, and the periodic table in chemistry a fraud.

The claim that the signatories were an 'independent consortium' was dubious for several reasons. First, there is the obvious investment in validating the authenticity of a controversial disorder for those 'who have devoted years, if not entire careers' to its study. In addition, many of the self-declared consortium of 'leading scientists' earn their incomes either through diagnosing and prescribing for ADHD or conducting drug-company funded research into the disorder.

British psychiatrist Sami Timimi believes the Consensus Statement was a response to the authors being 'shaken by criticism' of ADHD diagnosing and prescribing.[368] Timimi is highly critical of the Consensus Statement and sees it as an attempt to shut down debate:

> Not only is it completely counter to the spirit and practice of science to cease questioning the validity of ADHD as proposed by the consensus statement, there is an ethical and moral responsibility to do so. It is regrettable that they wish to close down debate prematurely and in a way not becoming of academics. The evidence shows that the debate is far from over.[369]

The authors of the Consensus Statement, according to Timimi, were 'well-known advocates of drug treatment for children with ADHD' who in the statement did 'not declare their financial interests and/or their links with pharmaceutical companies'.[370] The International Consensus Statement was an attempt by Barkley and its other authors to present the legitimacy of ADHD as an indisputable truth. Documents such as this have the effect of dumbing down debate by substituting prejudice for science. Despite the fundamentalist fervour of the authors, the fact is that ADHD is no more than a very loosely defined set of symptoms for which 'leading scientists' identify no cause and no cure and no evidence to support their assertion that 'ADHD is a real medical condition'.

The ironic thing is that ADHD could be 'cured' by consensus just as 'sexual deviation disorder' was cured. All we need to do is agree to stop believing in unproven theories about genetics and chemical imbalances causing children to be childlike. If we just let them be kids and gave them the time they need to grow up many children currently diagnosed with ADHD would be fine. Others would still have the problems that are currently contributing to their behaviour, but they wouldn't also have a stigmatising label and a daily amphetamine habit. Can you imagine how much kids would benefit from a consensus of adults agreeing that we will help children by finding out what is causing their problems and respond accordingly?

Sadly, there are no signs this is going to happen anytime soon. Instead the ADHD Industry will continue to offer a dumbed down label and drugs and justify its conduct through dodgy research. Most of the research undertaken by the proponents of ADHD, including the signatories of the International Consensus Statement, is designed to show either that ADHD medications alter behaviour in the short-term, or that children diagnosed with ADHD are different from other children.

Stimulants invariably appear more effective than non-drug treatments in short-term trials for two reasons. First, low dose amphetamines alter behaviour much faster than non-drug treatments, and improvement is usually measured by short-term symptom management, with drug trials often lasting for no longer than a few weeks. In addition, while the behaviour-altering effects of low dose psychostimulants are almost universal – narrowing focus in most people regardless of their 'ADHD' status – the effects of other forms of treatment are not. Diet modification, for example, may be of little or no benefit if the underlying cause of behavioural problems is severe family dysfunction.

The thousands of short-term studies confirming the behaviour altering effects of stimulants are in that sense valid. However, the many claims of new research purporting to prove biological differences have all been shown to be false or gross exaggerations of differences applying to only a small subset of children labelled ADHD. Many of these studies claimed to show differences between ADHD and non-ADHD brains, compared ADHD brains that had never been medicated, to ADHD brains that had been exposed to psychostimulants that have been shown to cause brain atrophy and retard growth.[371]

ADHD and Genetics

One of the biggest and most powerful deceptions ever in regard to ADHD occurred in September 2010 when the world media buzzed with the news that a group of British researchers had found the 'Holy Grail' for proponents of ADHD, by proving its genetic basis.[372] [373] [374] One of the researchers, Professor Anita Thapar of Cardiff University, proclaimed emphatically 'now we can say with confidence that ADHD is a genetic disease'.[375] Thapar's claim was nonsense, but by the time critics had identified the flaws in the research, the media circus had moved on and unknown millions of people around the globe had read, seen or heard the unchallenged proclamation that 'ADHD is a genetic disease'.

Professor Thapar's research is typical of the flawed science that supports ADHD. The study involved comparing the genetic codes of 366 children diagnosed with ADHD with those of 1047 'non-ADHD' control children. Thapar's research group found 13.9% (51) of children with ADHD had short lengths of their genetic code that were either duplicated or missing. This compared with 7.4% (78) of the 'control children'.[376] In other words, the vast majority of 'ADHD children' (86%) did not have the hypothesised 'ADHD genes' and some 'non-ADHD children' did.

Even the 13.9% to 7.4% difference is of questionable significance as there appears to be significant differences between the average IQ of the two groups. The mean recorded IQ of the 366 children 'with ADHD' was 86, fourteen points below the general population average of 100. Although the IQ of the 1047 'non-ADHD' children was not specified, presumably they were as intelligent as the general population. Furthermore, when 33 intellectually impaired 'ADHD children' (IQ lower than 70) were excluded from the ADHD cohort only 11% of the remaining 333 had the hypothesised ADHD genetic abnormality. Even with the intellectually impaired children removed, the average IQ (89) of the 333 remaining in the ADHD group was significantly lower than the control group (presumed to be 100). [377]

To be a valid comparison the study should have compared like with like. That is, the 'ADHD' cohort of children should have had the same average IQ as the 'non-ADHD' cohort of children. However the reason offered by the authors for not comparing like with like – being that they did not have IQ measures for the control group – was convenience not science. The authors offered the explanation that the low average IQ of the ADHD cohort was of no consequence as the non-ADHD cohort included 'individuals spanning a wide IQ spectrum which presumably includes those with a lower IQ'.[378]

This evidence is more suggestive of a weak relationship between the identified genetic abnormality and intellectual disadvantage than it is of ADHD. The authors of the study acknowledged the likely association between intellectual disability and the genetic abnormality identified but defended their comparisons of populations with a low average IQ with a normal control population. All of this, of course, was lost on the media. They reported Thapar's overblown, unsubstantiated conclusion as scientific fact, and failed to report the IQ differences between so called 'ADHD children' and normal children.

There have been, and will continue to be, many false dawns; where hyped claims like Thapar's are on closer inspection, shown to be false. It remains the case that no specific ADHD genes, or combination of genes, have been identified. The failure to identify specific genes is not caused by a lack of looking. Considerable research effort has been expended searching for the hypothesised genetic basis of ADHD.

Finding a genetic basis for ADHD would involve finding a genetic basis for inattentive and/or impulsive/hyperactive behaviour. Individual behavioural differences, like distractibility and hyperactivity, are in part determined by genetics, and twin and family studies have suggested a strong genetic component in ADHD type behaviours.[379] [380] But difference is not disease! So, even if researchers found consistent genetic or other biological diagnostic differences between people who consistently display

ADHD-like behaviours and those who don't, (e.g. those who like and dislike homework) that would not make ADHD a legitimate psychiatric disorder. As Queensland psychologist Bob Jacobs points out:

> There may be physiological differences between people who are right-handed and left-handed, or people who prefer the colour red over the colour blue. But it doesn't make either group 'sick'. We know that people have individual physical differences, but it is dangerous ground to say that those differences are a 'disorder', just because they are in the minority, or because they cause problems with fitting into society's rigid structures (like school).[381]

Yet despite Jacob's powerful argument, and the lack of rigorous evidence supporting its validity, or a scientific method of diagnosing the 'disease', ADHD is universally recognised by Western Government health authorities as a legitimate psychiatric 'disorder'. The obvious question is why has a hypothesis that ADHD is a 'genetic biochemical brain imbalance' achieved this status?

The core reason is that it suits so many stakeholders to believe in ADHD. The diagnosis offers a simple explanation, and psychostimulants a quick solution, to complex problems in time poor societies. Busy clinicians get a quick, easy, lucrative diagnosis and treatment. Struggling teachers get a compliant child. And governments get a cheap way of appearing to meet child mental health demands. In addition, many parents are irresistibly attracted to the promise of a quick fix. But in reality they are short-changing their child. The ADHD label lowers expectations of both the child and the adults in the child's life, and low expectations become a self-fulfilling prophecy.

ADHD and Drug Abuse

A common focus for ADHD Industry research is to show that left undiagnosed and untreated ADHD causes horrific life outcomes. Even criminality and drug abuse are attributed to undiagnosed, and therefore un-medicated, ADHD. An example is the following statement by ADHD 'expert' Professor David Coghill.

> Adults with ADHD that are untreated are much more likely to have problems with substance misuse, they are more likely to smoke and drink as well as take illegal drugs. They are much more likely to be involved in accidents, either as a pedestrian or as a driver of a vehicle, because of their impulsive behaviour. They are much more likely to be involved in criminal activity. They have more family breakups, so they are more likely to be divorced, to have difficulties in their family relationships.[382]

The effect of this association with extreme dysfunctional behaviour is to create a sense of crisis that extreme consequences will result from ADHD going untreated – which really means un-medicated. Criminal and drug-taking behaviour are in themselves dysfunctional and most often impulsive acts. How many drug addicts aren't forgetful, distracted or disorganised? It is self-evident that many criminals and drug addicts tend to demonstrate ADHD behaviours and certainly live dysfunctional lives, therefore qualifying for a diagnosis of adult ADHD. Yet to argue that ADHD, when left un-medicated, causes criminal behaviour or drug abuse is to confuse cause and effect. It involves identifying dysfunction in what is already identified as a dysfunctional population. This is the equivalent of being able to bet on a horse after the race has finished.

The claims that the ADHD Industry makes about treating the disorder and drug use are particularly absurd. Fundamentally they argue that unless we give children with challenging behaviours a daily amphetamine habit they will go onto become drug addicts. All ADHD stimulants are addictive and carry similar warnings for abuse to that below for Dexedrine, a brand of dexamphetamine.[383]

AMPHETAMINES HAVE A HIGH POTENTIAL FOR ABUSE. ADMINISTRATION OF AMPHETAMINES FOR PROLONGED PERIODS OF TIME MAY LEAD TO DRUG DEPENDENCE AND MUST BE AVOIDED. PARTICULAR ATTENTION SHOULD BE PAID TO THE POSSIBILITY OF SUBJECTS OBTAINING AMPHETAMINES FOR NON-THERAPEUTIC USE OR DISTRIBUTION TO OTHERS, AND THE DRUGS SHOULD BE PRESCRIBED OR DISPENSED SPARINGLY. MISUSE OF AMPHETAMINES MAY CAUSE SUDDEN DEATH AND SERIOUS CARDIO-VASCULAR ADVERSE EVENTS.

Even the American Psychiatric Association recognise that prescribed stimulants, methamphetamine, and cocaine are 'neuro-pharmacologically alike'.[384] DSM-5 recognises the abuse and addiction of these drugs in a common class of 'Stimulant Related Disorders'. It states: 'Prescribed stimulants may be diverted into the illegal market. The effects of amphetamines and amphetamine-like drugs are similar to those of cocaine, such that the criteria for stimulant use disorder are presented here as a single disorder.'[385]

Parents and patients rely on prescribing clinicians to heed such warnings, or, at the very least, pass them on and inform them of the risks. Too often this doesn't happen. Sometimes the consequences are devastating, even life-ending. Such was the case for Claire Murray.

RIP Claire Murray – a Victim of Perth's Generation deX

In 1998 Perth parents Mick and Val Murray took their twelve-year-old daughter Claire Murray to a paediatrician and prominent ADHD 'specialist' Dr Ken Whiting. Claire had been a bright and happy girl but Val and Mick were worried about recent changes in her behaviour and school performance. They were anxious to find out what was going on and were referred to Dr Whiting by their GP. Dr Whiting diagnosed Claire with ADHD at the first consultation and put her on a high dose of dexamphetamine. Claire disclosed many years later to Val and Mick that she had been sexually assaulted by an adult on a school camp and threatened if she told anybody. Below is an excerpt from a letter Mick wrote and asked me to read to the Western Australian Legislative Assembly in 2010 when Claire was seeking help from the Government to get a second liver transplant.

To Whom It May Concern

My daughter, Claire Rita Murray (DOB 14/3/85), is a heroin addict with three to six months to live. Claire was an A grade student at Ursula Frayne Catholic College until she was twelve years of age. At this time Claire was diagnosed with ADHD and introduced to her first drug dexamphetamine. Claire was prescribed 10mg of this drug four times a day for a period of eighteen months by her paediatrician, Dr Ken Whiting; and from that day on my daughter Claire and her family's problems began.

For the past twelve years Claire has had difficulties with everyday life, has been to every rehabilitation establishment in Perth. Throughout all this time she has been supported by her family. Claire was brought up in a loving family environment; has an older sister and a younger brother who both have successful careers and live healthy lives. Medical studies have shown that the treatment of ADHD at that time was misdiagnosed and that the drug was wrongly prescribed.

Unfortunately last September, while Claire was on a methadone program, her liver failed because of her past substance abuse. Claire was lucky enough to qualify for a liver transplant and was psychologically and physically deemed fit for a transplant.

The liver transplant was carried out at Sir Charles Gairdner Hospital on 6/9/09; however, there was a complication the following day that required a further operation to graft an artery. Claire spent the next three weeks in hospital and was eventually discharged.

Claire went well for a short time but unfortunately she still had her addiction and started to use drugs once again – which doctors believe was solely responsible for the failure of Claire's new liver... In my opinion my daughter's addiction is the result of being wrongly prescribed dexamphetamines and therefore I feel that the medical authorities should take full responsibility for her present condition.

Claire's original liver failed because of her drug addiction and she received a transplant in 2009. Within months of receiving the transplant Claire returned to abusing heroin and her donated liver failed. Mick and Val told me on multiple occasions they were never informed about the addictive nature of dexamphetamine.[386] In 2010 Claire's case became highly publicised when the Western Australian government provided a $250,000 interest-free loan to her family so that she could undergo a live liver transplant in Singapore. Claire's aunt Caroline courageously provided a partial liver donation and in March 2010 Claire and her aunt were operated on in Singapore.

Sadly, Claire's second transplant failed due to complications, and she died aged twenty-five in Singapore on 1 April 2010, surrounded by Mick, Val and other family members, but away from her two young children. Claire's tragic story was made into a damning documentary *Wild Butterfly*. One of the most shocking things to witness (that is highlighted in *Wild Butterfly*) was how Claire and her family were vilified by sections of the public and in the media. *60 Minutes* reporter

Liam Bartlett deserves special condemnation. He did a particularly nasty hatchet job on Claire when she was in Singapore.

I advocated for Claire at the time publicly trying to highlight that as a twelve-year-old Claire through no fault of hers or her family was given a high dose, daily amphetamine habit. I did not know when I was advocating for Claire that she had been sexually abused. Understandably Claire, Mick and Val wanted to keep that secret. Nonetheless, I mistakenly thought when the public understood how she was initially introduced to drugs they would be sympathetic. I was very wrong about that. Claire's vilification by some of my fellow West Australians was ugly, cruel and ignorant.

In the WA Parliament I briefly discussed the role Dr Whiting had played in not just in Claire's treatment but also in the regulation of ADHD prescribing in Western Australia. With hindsight I regret not fully using the protections parliamentary privilege afforded me when I had the opportunity. Well before I entered the WA state parliament in February 2001, I knew Dr Whiting. In fact, it is entirely accurate to say it was my experience of Dr Whiting when I was a teacher in Perth from 1995 to 2000 that was the catalyst for my 25-year involvement in the ADHD debate.

Dr Whiting wasn't just a frequent prescriber he was on the WA Health Department Stimulants Committee that was charged with making sure that responsible prescribing occurred. In my first book *Speed Up and Sit Still – the controversies of ADHD diagnosis and treatment* and in my PhD thesis I detailed how the Stimulants Committee failed to protect WA children like Claire. Put very politely, heavy prescribers were responsible for policing their own prescribing practices and the results were predictable.

Mick, Val, and their grandchildren (Claire's children) and their family still suffer. Dr Whiting is (as at July 2020) Patron of ADHD WA (previously called the Learning and Attentional Disorders Society or LADS). If Australia had stronger freedom of speech protections I would risk being less polite about Dr Whiting and LADS.

Western Australia's Unique ADHD History

Claire's story is just one chapter in the ongoing story about ADHD in Western Australia. WA has a unique history as the world's first ADHD hotspot to see a massive decrease in ADHD child prescribing rates (50% drop between 2002 and 2008).[387] However, over the last decade there has been a significant rebound. So it is a history in three parts: a period of rapidly rising prescribing rates, followed by a massive decline, and then a strong rebound.

The Rise 1993-2002: Throughout the 1990s the proportion of children and adolescents (aged 0 to 17) prescribed Amphetamine Type Stimulants grew more rapidly in WA than elsewhere in Australia. By 2000 prescribing rates were approximately 2.8 times the average of other Australian states and were among the highest in the world. They grew a further 15% between 2000 and 2002.[388]

The Fall 2003-10: Following significant regulatory reforms prescribing rates for 0 to 17-year-olds declined and by 2010 were approximately halved. [389] [390] During this period child and adolescent prescribing rates rose rapidly in all other states. By 2011 WA rates were approximately 11% below the national average.

The Rebound 2011 onwards: There was a rebound from 1.05% (in 2010) to 1.62% in 2017. Most of the growth occurred between 2014 and 2017, when there was a jump from 6,971 to 9,587 (a 37.5% rise) in the number of 0 to 17-year-olds receiving prescribed ATS despite the WA population only increasing by 4%.[391]

Throughout the 1990s and early 2000s in Western Australia there was considerable anecdotal reporting of the diversion of ADHD amphetamines amongst WA teenagers and young adults. When data became available through the *Australian Secondary Students' Alcohol and Drug Survey* (ASSAD) these suspicions were confirmed. ASSAD surveys indicated a reduction in 'last 12 month amphetamine abuse' by 12-17-year-olds from 10.3% in 2002 to 5.1% in 2008.[392] This 51% reduction in self-reported abuse occurred over a similar time period as the 50% fall in ADHD child stimulant prescribing rates.

Even though prescription rates had begun to drop by 2005, the ASSAD survey estimated that 9,492 (5.5%) of Western Australia's secondary school students had abused prescription ADHD amphetamines in the last year. The same survey found that amongst 12-17-year-olds, 84% of those who had abused amphetamines in the last year had abused diverted stimulants, and that 27% of those who had been prescribed stimulant medication either gave it away or sold it. It also showed that 45% of Western Australian high school students who had ever taken dexamphetamine or methylphenidate were not prescribed the drugs by a doctor.[393]

Despite the clear evidence of significant abuse of prescription amphetamines in the 2005 ASSAD survey, it wasn't until 2017 that secondary school students were surveyed again. Even then it was only about dexamphetamine abuse, and only in WA. The 2017 ASSAD surveyed 3,361 WA secondary students about their non-medical use of dexamphetamine – 3% reported non-medical use in the last 12 months.[394] In comparison, approximately 1.2% were prescribed dexamphetamine. This indicates that for every WA secondary school student prescribed dexamphetamine approximately 2.5 used it non-medically.

The 3% figure does not include those students who had non-medically used Ritalin or other brands of methylphenidate. In 2017 dexamphetamine was only prescribed to about 40% of WA children who took an ADHD drug.[395] It is therefore likely that the rate of last

12-month non-medical use of all forms of prescribed ADHD drugs was much higher than 3%. It is clear that Claire Murray was not an isolated case. Over the last twenty years unknown tens of thousands of WA adolescents have abused prescription ADHD amphetamines.

WA adults have long been prescribed ADHD stimulants at many times the rates of adults in other states. In 2002 they were prescribed PBS dexamphetamine (until 2005 the only PBS-subsidised ATS) at over seven times the rate of other Australian adults.[396] By 2008, all stimulant medications were PBS-sponsored and there was a narrowing of the gap. However, in 2017 WA adults were still over 2.6 times more likely than other Australian adults to receive PBS-subsidised Amphetamine Type Stimulant for ADHD. [397] WA has also consistently reported high rates of meth/amphetamine use compared to other Australian states and there is evidence from multiple sources that indicates dexamphetamine abuse is a significant part of WA's amphetamine abuse culture.

Far from supporting the ADHD Industry assertion that medication use prevents illicit drug abuse by self-medicating untreated ADHD sufferers, the WA experience is that there is a positive correlation between amphetamine abuse rates and the legal prescribing rates for amphetamines for the treatment of ADHD. This supports the commonsense proposition that prescribing amphetamines facilitates the abuse of amphetamines. Nonetheless, ADHD proponents continue to push children towards ADHD amphetamines using the rationale that in doing so they prevent future drug abuse.

The Emperor's New Disorder

Proponents of ADHD deserve ridicule for this and so many of their other absurd claims. Ultimately they are arguing that losing your toys, playing too loudly, interrupting etc. are evidence of a biochemical brain imbalance, and that amphetamines are good for children and prevent drug abuse. It is nonsense propped up by lies and faulty analysis, like that produced by Professor Thapar.

In summary, the lies told about ADHD and the effects of ADHD 'medications' combine to produce a self-fulfilling prophecy of failure, dysfunction and drug abuse. The addictive properties of amphetamines, and the likely long term adverse effects of 'medications', combined with the short-term cycle of temporary compliant behaviour and withdrawal symptoms, are all mistakenly attributed to the 'patient's' ADHD rather than the label and the drugs. This reinforces the ongoing need for the same label and drugs that have created, or at best exacerbated, existing problems.

What a dishonest but wonderfully profitable marketing circle this is for the ADHD drug manufacturers! What a terrible future it is for so many children completely powerless to prevent their adult imposed 'diagnosis and drug' downwards spiral of expectation, performance and addiction!

Breaking this cycle and ending the ADHD fraud requires leadership. It requires prominent people in psychiatry, psychology, politics, popular culture and the media to say that the ADHD Emperors have no clothes. The problem to date has been that, even in extreme cases – like when Harvard Professor Joseph Biederman[398] was caught accepting drug company kick-backs – ADHD gurus get to keep their money, power and prestige, and their corrupted research continues to influence clinical practice.

ADHD critics need to be bolder, organised, and call a spade a spade. ADHD proponents have had every opportunity to validate their claims and the best they can come up with are lies and quarter truths supported by pseudoscience. The time for talking about ADHD being misdiagnosed and overmedicated has passed. It is time to start telling the whole inconvenient truth. ADHD is a fraud and this truth needs to be proclaimed loudly and often.

Chapter 7

Professor Ian Hickie: Australia's Depression Salesman-Scientist.

This Chapter was prepared with the assistance of Dr Melissa Raven

Ian Hickie is a Professor of Psychiatry and Co-Director, Health and Policy, at the University of Sydney's *Brain and Mind Centre*. In 2000, he was the inaugural CEO of beyondblue, a position he held until September 2003, when he commenced as Professor of Psychiatry and inaugural Executive Director of the *Brain and Mind Research Institute* (renamed the Brain and Mind Centre in 2015). He is an NHMRC Senior Principal Research Fellow (2013-2017 and 2018-22), having previously been an inaugural NHMRC Australian Fellow (2008-12). He was an inaugural Commissioner on Australia's *National Mental Health Commission* (2012-18) and was a founding board member of *headspace* (2006 to 2012)[399]. Professor Hickie has authored or co-authored over 500 peer-reviewed articles[400]. He and his life partner, and frequent research partner, psychiatrist Dr Elizabeth Scott, have received financial support from multiple pharmaceutical companies, particularly earlier in his career. He is the Chief Scientific Advisor to, and a 5% equity shareholder in, InnoWell, a company that was formed by the University of Sydney and PricewaterhouseCoopers (PwC) to deliver the $30 million Australian Government-funded 'Project Synergy' – a three-year program to develop innovative digital technologies for use in mental health services – and is now expanding its services.

Professor Ian Hickie and Professor Patrick McGorry are frequent allies, often selling the same core message. Both are charismatic and work the media extremely well. Both are well connected to politicians and bureaucrats, and speak authoritatively, claiming in-depth expertise in relation to a broad range of mental health issues. However, their demeanours are often different.

McGorry's 'propaganda' dummy-spit in response to the journal article that Melissa Raven, Jon Jureidini and I wrote, that was critical of his advice about antidepressants and youth suicide (see Chapter 4), was unusual. More often he is the diplomat, charming his critics by focusing on points of agreement, or creating the impression of consensus even where there is none. McGorry typically shares his insights with you politely. He often acknowledges the concerns of critics and reassures them that the issues have been considered and dealt with. He makes his target audience feel as if they already intuitively know the truths that he shares with them. McGorry is brilliant at politely damning governments with faint praise, often thanking them for increased funding for headspace or another of his programs but making it clear that much more funding is required.

In contrast, Hickie is the assertive warrior, more combative; sometimes confronting or dismissing his critics aggressively. Hickie dares doubters to be foolish enough to disagree.

My first experience of Hickie, in 2010, left me wondering how thoroughly he researched issues he was prepared to offer expert commentary on. It related to the Raine Study ADHD Drug Review (discussed briefly in Chapter 6). Speaking on ABC Radio's PM Program, Hickie minimised the significance of the key finding of the research: that past stimulant use increased the probability of an ADHD diagnosed child falling behind at school by a massive 950%.[401]

This finding undermined the hypothetical basis of medicating for ADHD, namely that if you don't medicate (i.e. drug with amphetamines) your 'disordered' child, you are dooming them to a lifetime of academic and career underachievement. Hickie, who had no involvement in the Raine ADHD research, explained away this key finding, saying that 'typically those kids who go on the medication are considerably worse to start with'.[402]

I was a member of the committee that commissioned the research. Initially, the ADHD medication proponents on that committee tried to claim that the reason the outcomes for the medicated children were worse than those for the unmedicated children was most probably because the medicated children had more severe ADHD – the same argument Hickie used. However, I insisted on a comparison of the groups at age five, which was prior to any of the children having been medicated. This analysis established that there were no statistically significant differences in developmental, behavioural and health measures before the children were medicated. This was made clear in the study, but it was not reflected in Hickie's comments.

Even if Hickie's comments had been valid, and the children who had been medicated were 'considerably worse to start with', if stimulants were effective in the long term, those children should have been performing at least as well at school – and not failing at 10.5 times the rate – as those with moderate, unmedicated ADHD.

Subsequent to this experience, I have observed Hickie's comments on a range of issues. In my opinion, he speaks persuasively, often forcefully, on just about anything and everything related to mental health.

As discussed in Chapter 5, many Australian politicians, from prime ministers down, have been heavily influenced by, and even deferential to, Hickie and McGorry. In my view, this is largely because much of the mainstream media, particularly the ABC (see Chapter 8), have persistently portrayed them as visionary mental health leaders. But it is also because mental health is such a mysterious policy area for non-experts that the certainty offered by seemingly authoritative voices like Hickie's is attractive to time-pressured and confused journalists and politicians.

Hickie and Beyond Blue

As briefly discussed in Chapter 4, Hickie first became increasingly prominent in the national mental health arena in October 2000 when he became the inaugural CEO of beyondblue – the national depression initiative (rebranded Beyond Blue circa 2018). He held the position until September 2003, when he commenced as Professor of Psychiatry and inaugural Executive Director of the Brain and Mind Research Institute (BMRI) at the University of Sydney. After commencing at BMRI, Hickie was Clinical Advisor to Beyond Blue from 2003 to 2006, during which time he continued to champion the organisation and its mission.[403] [404] [405]

Initial funding of $37 million over five years was secured by Beyond Blue in 2000, with the Commonwealth and Victorian Governments contributing $17.5 million each, with much smaller contributions from the governments of South Australian, Australian Capital Territory, Northern Territory, and Tasmania.[406]

In a media release announcing the Australian Government support for Beyond Blue, Dr Michael Wooldridge, the Howard Government's

Health Minister, declared:

> Beyond Blue will turn the Depression Initiative's ideas into
> actions. The World Health Organisation has predicted that by
> the year 2020 depression will be the world's second largest health
> problem behind heart disease.[407]

It appears that, for Beyond Blue, having depression recognised by
the year 2020 as Australia's second largest health problem has been an
aspirational goal.

Together with Hickie and Woolridge, former Victorian Liberal Premier
Jeff Kennett was instrumental in garnering political support for Beyond
Blue.[408] Before losing the 1999 Victorian state election, Kennett had
become very concerned about the problem of young male suicide in
rural Victoria, and he started to speak publicly about it. Kennett's suicide
prevention campaign rapidly attracted bipartisan support, transcending
divisions between the two main political forces in Australian politics.
This bipartisan support continues today and has created some unusual
alliances. Kennett, a doyen of the Liberal Party, was Chairperson of
Beyond Blue from 2000 until 2017, when he retired and publicly anointed
former Labor Prime Minister Julia Gillard as his successor.

Beyond Blue has scaled up massively since its inception. In recent
years, it has broadened its remit to include anxiety and other related
mental disorders. In the 2019 financial year, it had annual revenue of
over $60 million, with the Commonwealth Government contributing
over $39.4 million, the States and Territories nearly $5.2 million,
and most of the rest coming from donations. As at 30 June 2019, the
organisation had net assets of over $55 million.[409]

Pharmaceutical industry-funded depression awareness campaigns
have played a major role in the popularisation of depression worldwide,
but Beyond Blue has been the most visible force behind depression's
remarkable rise to prominence in Australia. Beyond Blue is widely

accepted as the national authority on depression. This is manifest in the fact that media reports about depression, suicide, and related topics very often end with contact details for Beyond Blue.

Although it has never accepted pharmaceutical company funding, Beyond Blue has been a strong advocate for the orthodox story about depression and antidepressants, i.e. that depression is common, serious, and treatable, and that antidepressants reduce the risk of suicide. With Beyond Blue's promotion, this orthodox story has dominated media coverage.

There can be little doubt that, like Suicide Prevention Australia (see Chapter 4), Beyond Blue has prospered at the same time as prescribing and suicide rates have soared. Its activities have undoubtedly contributed to the massive rise in rates of depression and anxiety diagnosis and antidepressant prescribing. Clearly, in terms of influence and organisation growth, Beyond Blue has been an extraordinary success. Whether it has helped ordinary Australians is another question.

In 2004, Hickie suggested that Beyond Blue had been more successful than the UK Defeat Depression Campaign:

> To date, few countries in the developed world have attempted such a coordinated population health response to the burden of depression. The most recent British initiative achieved limited benefits. Improvements of 5%-10% were reported in terms of more positive attitudes to depression, reported experiences of depression, attitudes to antidepressants and treatment from GPs. Few GPs (11%) had definitely made changes in their management of depression as a result of the campaign. At this early stage, the Australian experience appears to be achieving wider benefits and establishing a broader framework for more sustainable changes in community attitudes and health service reform.[410]

Clearly Hickie regarded the popularisation of depression as an indicator of success. However, this approach has attracted criticism, most notably from Professor Gordon Parker, who was the Director of the Black Dog Institute at the University of New South Wales. Hickie and Parker are former colleagues but, as detailed in the *Sydney Morning Herald* in 2004, they have engaged in strident public disagreement.

Extract from **It's professors at 10 paces as drugs row gets personal**[411]

Julie Robotham, *Sydney Morning Herald*, June 26, 2004.
A ferocious wrangle has erupted between two of Sydney's most prominent psychiatrists over the profession's latest high-profile issue – are antidepressant drugs effective? The protagonists are the polar opposites of psychiatry. Gordon Parker is the old-school professor with the intense gaze and the patrician manner. Ian Hickie is the hyperactive moderniser; a gregarious salesman of mental health to a sceptical community.

Complicating the argument is the fact that Hickie studied under Parker as an undergraduate at the University of NSW. In a pair of articles littered with academic insults, each has savaged the scientific basis of the other's work and levelled accusations of working against patients' interests. Their dispute comes amid a swell of public demand for reassurance about the use of new antidepressants after a decade of surging prescriptions since Prozac first hit the market. Reports have emerged that the drugs may trigger psychosis, and concern has grown that they can trigger suicide in adolescents.

… Parker says the category of 'major depression', for which many of the drugs were tested, is not a true diagnosis but a catch-all promoted by manufacturers. As well, the 'pristine' patients in clinical trials are unlike those who need medication in real life, where serious depression is usually complicated by drugs, alcohol, other illnesses or personality traits.

Hickie counter-attacks in the same journal, saying his colleague's views are insubstantial and threaten to 'set back the scientific basis of clinical psychiatry and further undermine our public credibility'. 'Consumers and their families might rightly be distressed by this view, especially when it is expressed by such an eminent clinician,' he writes. Exhaustive research, including trials comparing antidepressants with placebos, were especially vital for psychiatry, Hickie said in an interview. This was because 'ours is an area ripe for exploitation of patients', where unproven therapies and cult practitioners could readily get traction among the vulnerable.

Hickie defended the strident language of his rebuttal, saying it was not personal and that he had a responsibility to balance the picture presented by Parker. Hickie slipped quietly from the University of NSW to the University of Sydney last year after his high-profile term as head of the national depression initiative, beyondblue. The move gives him more distance from his former mentor, and emphasises their divisions. Hickie says that he and Parker are 'mutually polite' whenever they meet while Parker describes the relationship as 'very amiable'.[412]

This was not a one-off disagreement. In 2001, Hickie was lead author of a paper[413] that criticised a 2000 paper by Parker that stated: 'Depression can be a normal mood state – brief, self-remitting, and ubiquitous'.[414] Parker in turn has repeatedly publicly decried the fact that the diagnosis and treatment of depression has been 'dumbed down'.[415]

Irrespective of Parker's criticisms, it is undeniable that Hickie's initial leadership of Beyond Blue worked well both for him and for the organisation. Hickie rapidly developed a high profile in the media, and he was appointed to numerous government and NGO committees, boards, and working groups, giving him considerable influence over mental health policy. In 2006, Hickie was named by the *Australian Financial Review* as one of the Australia's top 10 cultural influencers.[416] At the time, he was the psychiatrist most likely to be approached by the Australian media for comment on any mental health issue, and one of very few psychiatrists whose name was familiar to many Australians other than mental health professionals.

Beyond Blue and the SPHERE project

In the late 1990s, Hickie and his life and research partner, psychiatrist Dr Elizabeth Scott, developed SPHERE: the national depression project.[417] SPHERE was a general practitioner depression diagnosis and treatment training program, co-ordinated by Scott.[418] Although the SPHERE project provided GPs with training in cognitive behavioural therapy, it promoted antidepressant prescribing as being integral to the treatment of depression.

Initially, SPHERE received funding from Bristol Myers Squibb, as well as the Australian and New South Wales governments.[419] Hickie had also done work for other pharmaceutical companies, but when he was appointed by Beyond Blue, he declared that he would no longer be undertaking such work.[420]

In 2000, shortly after Hickie's commencement as CEO, Beyond Blue turned down $1.2 million funding from Pfizer – the manufacturer of Zoloft® (sertraline), a blockbuster SSRI antidepressant.[421] Hickie later claimed that he was instrumental in refusing Pfizer's offer.[422] However, a few months after Beyond Blue rejected the drug company's offer, Pfizer became a SPHERE implementation partner,[423] reportedly because Pfizer was 'keen to lift their activity and make up lost ground' to a rival antidepressant, Effexor.[424]

According to her CV on the BMRI website, Scott was the coordinator of the SPHERE General Practitioner training Program until at least 2008.[425] She had also set up several interlinked business entities that were involved in the SPHERE project, including Educational Health Solutions (registered in 1996) and Devine Publishing (registered in 1997).[426] Educational Health Solutions was taken over by Strange & Partners Pty Ltd in 2000.[427] Nine days later, former pharmaceutical company executive Shane Duncan became a Director of Strange & Partners.[428] Later, by 2007, Duncan had merged Educational Health Solutions into a new business entity called Lifeblood.[429]

In July 2001, Beyond Blue published a 58-page glossy supplement about the SPHERE project, funded by the Australian Government (i.e. taxpayers) in the *Medical Journal of Australia*.[430] The supplement presented SPHERE in a very favourable light, starting with the National Mental Health Strategy and Beyond Blue logos on the front cover. It highlighted the results of a survey, using Hickie's Somatic and Psychological HEalth REport (SPHERE) questionnaire, which suggested that depression was massively under-recognised and under-treated. Both the questionnaire and the survey results have been strongly criticised.[431] [432]

The SPHERE questionnaire includes items related to physical discomfort and stress, without excluding physical and circumstantial causes. Its use can result in people being flagged as suffering a mental disorder on the basis of evidence as slight as reporting muscle pain after activity 'a good part of the time' and tired muscles after activity 'most of the time' over the past few weeks, or reporting being unable to overcome difficulties most of the time 'over the past few weeks'.[433]

The content of the SPHERE questionnaire is similar to that of the PRIME-MD questionnaire developed in the USA for Pfizer, which owns the copyright.[434] Both include many questions about somatic symptoms such as tiredness and pain.

The full SPHERE questionnaire is a 34-item questionnaire developed by Hickie and colleagues in the late 1990s. Often the shorter SPHERE-12 questionnaire, a 12-item version, is used. It comprises six items about psychological distress and six items about physical distress.[435]

SPHERE-12 questionnaire

Over the past few weeks have you been troubled by:	
Score: 0 = never or some of the time; 1 = a good part of the time; 2 = most of the time	
PSYCH-6 items	**SOMA-6 items**
☐ Feeling nervous or tense	☐ Muscle pain after activity
☐ Feeling unhappy and depressed	☐ Needing to sleep longer
☐ Feeling constantly under strain	☐ Prolonged tiredness after activity
☐ Everything getting on top of you	☐ Poor sleep
☐ Losing confidence	☐ Poor concentration
☐ Being unable to overcome difficulties	☐ Tired muscles after activity

To qualify as having a mental disorder, patients need to score a total of 2 or more on the PSYCH-6 items and/or 3 or more on the SOMA-6 items.

If a patient reports that they had experienced *one* of the PSYCH-6 problems 'most of the time' or two of them 'a good part of the time' in the past few weeks, they would score 2 on the PSYCH-6 scale. This means that someone who was stressed by work or family circumstances and felt unable to overcome difficulties 'a good part of the time' would qualify as having a mental disorder.

Alternatively, and even more bizarrely, if they reported that they had experienced muscle pain, prolonged tiredness, and tired muscles after activity 'a good part of the time', or one of them 'most of the time' and another one 'a good part of the time', after heavy exercise in the past few weeks, they would qualify as mentally disordered using the SOMA-6 scale.

These extraordinarily broad diagnostic criteria are reflected in a startling statistic. The final paper in the supplement concluded that 'Sixty-three percent of people attending general practice have some evidence of mental disorder'.[436] This claim was also included in the summary of the SPHERE project findings published in the Beyond Blue-funded *GP Review*.[437] It also generated some alarmist newspaper headlines, including '60pc of GPs' patients mentally ill' and 'Six in 10 GP patients have mental illness: study'.[438] [439]

The SPHERE project was also promoted in the *Depression Awareness Journal*, which was edited by controversial Victorian psychiatrist Professor Graham Burrows and was sponsored by multiple antidepressant manufacturers.[440] Burrows, whose reckless prescribing practices were later exposed by TV station Channel 7,[441] wrote at least three favourable editorial pieces about SPHERE.[442] In addition, several articles co-authored by Hickie, some promoting the SPHERE project were published in the journal.[443]

The *Depression Awareness Journal* also featured a case study of a woman who presented with fatigue and recurrent vaginal candidiasis. The case study promoted SPHERE's use not only as a diagnostic tool but also as a method of persuading a patient to accept a psychiatric diagnosis:

> Using the SPHERE self-report format, she was more willing to accept a psychological interpretation of her difficulties. After making the connection between her psychological state and her physical symptoms, she was able to move on to a more thorough psychological evaluation, and thus relevant treatments.[444]

The commentary in the case study stated that patients with depression 'usually emphasise the physical rather than psychological symptoms of their disorder'.[445] This fits well with the theme of somatisation (classifying physical symptoms as evidence of mental illness) promoted by Hickie through the SPHERE project[446] and in journal articles.[447] Despite the disease-mongering inherent in regarding physical symptoms as evidence of mental illness, SPHERE was enthusiastically embraced by many players.

The SPHERE supplement in the *Medical Journal of Australia* was funded by the Australian Department of Health and Aged Care.[448] In fact, 'funding to support the development and publication of a 50-page supplement to *The Medical Journal of Australia* on Sphere: a National Depression Project' was celebrated as a key achievement under the National Mental Health Strategy.[449]

In addition, Beyond Blue funded 'aspects of the SPHERE Project' and distribution of SPHERE educational materials to GPs:

> beyondblue has supported a variety of direct educational
> initiatives (e.g. through regular articles in *GP review*) as well as
> provision of educational materials to GPs for use in their clinical
> management of patients with depression and anxiety. These have
> included materials produced previously as part of the SPHERE
> Project as well as other materials specifically relevant to the
> practice of non-pharmacological forms of treatment.[450]

Many SPHERE materials were incorporated into the Beyond Blue website. Hickie was editorial director of Beyond Blue until at least 2006, several years after finishing up as CEO.[451] Some SPHERE materials remained on the Beyond Blue website for many years.[452]

Six years after the SPHERE supplement was published in the *Medical Journal of Australia*, the SPHERE project was trumpeted by Lifeblood as a highly successful Zoloft® marketing strategy for Pfizer:

> In 2001 Pfizer Australia joined SPHERE as an implementation
> partner. This partnership saw the SPHERE project offered
> to all Australian GPs. Through the implementation of the
> SPHERE training modules, the Pfizer sales team gained regular,
> unprecedented access to these key GPs, who had significant

interest in mental health. This activity assisted in restoring the market share and growth of the Pfizer antidepressant Zoloft®, restoring it to the Number One product in this market.[453]

That statement was in a 'Medical Education' case study on the website of Lifeblood, an offshoot of Educational Health Solutions, a company that Scott registered in 1996.[454] [455] Hickie also acknowledged, in 2009, the unusual marketing success of Zoloft® stating it had been a 'standout drug in Australia, though it hasn't been elsewhere in the world'.[456]

In effect, after refusing Pfizer's $1.2 million funding offer, Beyond Blue, led by Hickie, used National Mental Health Strategy funding from the Department of Health and Aged Care to pay for promotion of the SPHERE project, which boosted sales of Pfizer's blockbuster antidepressant Zoloft®.

Lifeblood's website also bragged about the business's 'close collaboration with government', its key opinion leader engagement, and its partnerships with the Hickie-led Brain & Mind Research Institute (BMRI) that provided 'unique access to some of Australia's leading neuroscience clinicians and researchers'.[457]

This boast was removed from the Lifeblood website in June 2010 (but is still available through web archives) shortly before the publication of an article in *The Australian* titled *GP jaunts 'boosted' drug sales.*[458] Around this time, Hickie's CV was also altered, deleting the following paragraph from his Career Overview:

Professor Hickie and colleagues established 'SPHERE: A National Depression Project'... In 1999, the SPHERE Project was awarded a Gold THEMHS Award for education and training in mental health in Australasia. This work now continues through an academic-commercial partnership (between the BMRI and Educational Health Solutions) based at the BMRI in Sydney. Currently, education and training modules in general practice education, related to psychological skills, bipolar disorder, early psychosis and development of collaborative care models, are in operation throughout Australia.[459]

Note* Educational Health Solutions had been incorporated into Lifeblood by the time Hickie wrote this.

In 2010 Lifeblood's website boasted that SPHERE had 'reached over 12,000 general practitioners nationally', roughly 40% of all Australian GPs.[460] When asked about the perception of conflict of interest between Pfizer's commercial interests and its role in medical education, Lifeblood managing director Shane Duncan told *The Australian*:

> I can see how you may interpret it that way but we're very comfortable we've been able to maintain distance between the content of the program and the marketing...They do logistics, and marketing of the program, which includes inviting GPs, paying for the meeting facilities or restaurants, those sort of things.[461]

Duncan added that Pfizer became a partner in SPHERE because the company was 'keen to lift their activity and make up [Zoloft's] lost ground' to a rival antidepressant Effexor, and that Lifeblood approached Pfizer because it was thought it would help build the drug company's 'credibility'.[462]

Hickie has on occasions not disclosed relevant financial links to the SPHERE project. However, in 2003, he declared he had 'received research funding and honoraria in the last five years from several pharmaceutical companies for conduct of General Practice training programs, notably SPHERE: A National Depression Project'.[463] During his tenure as Beyond Blue CEO, Educational Health Solutions (later Lifeblood) published numerous SPHERE training manuals and CDs co-authored by Hickie and Scott.[464] The development of these training materials was funded by Pfizer.[465]

Hickie's advocacy of SPHERE continued long after he left Beyond

Blue. The Brain and Mind Research Institute (BMRI), headed by Hickie, had an ongoing commercial relationship with SPHERE, and Lifeblood's Sydney office was located within the BMRI and 'doctors employed by the institute [BRMI] are [were] paid to review the medical content of SPHERE'.[466]

In 2010, in an article in *Australasian Psychiatry*, Hickie and his co-author Sebastian Rosenberg criticised both the Better Access program and the evaluation process commissioned by the Department of Health and Ageing. They highlighted the strengths of the SPHERE project, suggesting that SPHERE data could be used in the evaluation.[467] They argued that a 'genuine' evaluation of Better Access would include assessment of identification rates of psychological disorders in GP attendees; prevalence of all mental health treatments; demographic, professional and practice system data; impacts of treatments; and consumer experiences of care. They then outlined how the SPHERE project could provide answers to all these key questions.

In summary, SPHERE was set up by Hickie and Scott in Sydney in the 1990s. It followed them to Melbourne when Hickie was appointed CEO of Beyond Blue, and SPHERE was promoted by Beyond Blue in a glossy 58-page *Medical Journal of Australia* supplement paid for by Australian taxpayers. SPHERE then followed Hickie and Scott back to Sydney when Hickie was appointed as Executive Director of the Brain and Mind Research Institute at the University of Sydney. The BMRI then partnered with Educational Health Solutions/Lifeblood to promote SPHERE, and Pfizer eventually benefitted from increased sales of Zoloft®.

Although Beyond Blue did not accept pharmaceutical company funds, and Hickie said he would not take drug company funds while at Beyond Blue, the relationships between Hickie, Scott, Beyond Blue, SPHERE, Educational Health Solutions/Lifeblood, the Brain and Mind Research Institute and Pfizer were complex and opaque.

It is not clear how taxpayers, who funded both Beyond Blue and SPHERE, benefitted from a program that, among other things, promoted muscle pain and tiredness after activity as evidence of mental illness. It is, however, crystal clear that Pfizer profited.

Beyond Ageing Project – trialling antidepressants on the un-depressed!

In 2011, Hickie and other researchers at the Brain and Mind Research Institute, and research partners from Orygen and the Black Dog Institute, began recruiting participants in the Beyond Ageing Project Phase 2 – a trial comparing sertraline (the generic name for Zoloft®), fish-oil and placebo as a means of preventing older people (60+) from developing depression.[468] Hickie and his colleagues argued that the trial participants were at risk of major depression because of mildly elevated levels of psychological distress.

Professor of Psychiatry Jon Jureidini and Melissa Raven, together with two senior ethicists and a senior research psychologist, submitted a detailed complaint to the University of Sydney in December 2011 about the sertraline arm of the trial. They claimed that participants in the trial were given misleading information in the participant information sheet that exaggerated the potential benefits and minimised the potential harms of sertraline.

The risks associated with antidepressants – particularly for older people, who are often taking other drugs that can interact with antidepressants – include dizziness (which can cause falls and hip fracture) and strokes.[469] Jureidini, Raven and the other complainants also objected to the fact that no provision was made for follow-up at the end of the trial, despite the risk of withdrawal symptoms.

As a result of the complaint, participants were provided with a revised information sheet, and the consent process was repeated. However, the complainants were refused a copy of the new version and therefore were unable to assess whether participants received appropriate and accurate information.

The research received $448,634 in funding from the Bupa Health Foundation.[470] Hickie was a medical advisor to Bupa. This information was not included in the original information sheet. Also not disclosed were the BMRI's financial links with Pfizer, the largest manufacturer of sertraline, via the SPHERE academic-commercial partnership with Educational Health Solutions/Lifeblood.[471] It is also unclear whether the revised information sheet contained information about these or other potential conflicts of interest.

In 2015 – four years after recruiting for the trial commenced – Hickie and his fellow researchers argued that the research was needed 'to evaluate the role of neurobiological agents in preventing depressive symptoms in older populations at risk of depression... [with] interventions... targeted to the pathophysiology of disease'. They asserted that 'regardless of the effect size of treatment, the outcomes will offer major scientific advances regarding the neurobiological action of these agents'.[472]

However, in 2011 – in response to a comprehensive review that highlighted significant risks associate with antidepressant use by the elderly[473] – Hickie wrote an editorial, *Antidepressants in elderly people,* that stated 'we need to be clearer that drugs should not be recommended as first line treatments for less severe depressive disorders, particularly in older patients'. He further cautioned that 'given the potential harms, the decision to prescribe for an older person with depression should not be taken lightly'.[474] It is very puzzling that Hickie wrote this around the time that the Beyond Ageing Project trial was beginning, and participants were being told that 'this dose of sertraline is safe, well tolerated, and useful for improving mood', and 'Taking part in the study is considered to be of low risk. It is anticipated that participants will NOT experience any significant side effects'.[475]

When it's Hickie v. Hickie: Which Ian Hickie should we believe?

Reconciling Hickie's leadership of a drug trial of antidepressant use by older people to supposedly prevent depression, and his call for restraint in the use of antidepressants in older people with depression is difficult. However, it is just one example of Hickie espousing what appear to be contradictory positions. Despite his strongly expressed opinions, Hickie has been strikingly inconsistent in his position on multiple issues, including the relationship between electroconvulsive therapy (ECT) and retrograde amnesia (RA) – loss of long-term memory. RA is an acknowledged side effect of ECT but opinions are polarised about how persistent it can be.[476] [477]

Hickie was a co-author of an article published in January 2010 in the *Journal of Affective Disorders* titled *Electroconvulsive therapy-induced persistent retrograde amnesia: could it be minimised by ketamine or other pharmacological approaches?* The article appropriately acknowledged that 'available evidence indicates that ECT is objectively associated with persistent RA, and both clinicians and patients report that RA is distressing for patients'. It outlined several hypotheses for the relationship but stated that 'The mechanism for ECT-induced RA is unclear'.[478]

The paper concluded that the problem of ECT-induced RA was *'common, significant and undesirable'* and that it warranted exploration of other treatment methods. These potential treatment methods included experimenting with simultaneous administration of ketamine or other pharmacological approaches to see if this prevented the memory loss.

> Selective physical treatments for depression, such as transcranial magnetic stimulation, magnetic seizure therapy, vagus nerve stimulation, and transcranial direct current stimulation *[might]*

achieve an antidepressant effect without the cognitive side effects of generalised physical therapies such as ECT. However, it is possible that there is a simpler solution to the problem, and trialling ketamine for reducing ECT-induced RA would seem a cogent next step forward.[479]

Eleven months later, however, Hickie emphatically told The Age that the findings of a newly published review article[480] critical of the long-term effects of ECT 'were "ridiculous" and that while previously it was presumed that ECT caused memory loss, advances in brain imaging had shown the patient's depression was often to blame'. Furthermore, he asserted: 'This review is completely out of step with the last decade of systematic neuroscience and related clinical studies'.[481]

There were no Eureka-moment breakthroughs in brain imaging of people with depression between November 2009 (when the 2010 article was resubmitted and accepted) and December 2010 that could account for Hickie's massive about-turn. In addition, Hickie's co-authored article did not suggest that persistent ECT-induced memory loss was caused by patients' depression.

Hickie is not alone, in that many psychiatrists support the use of ECT, and it is not unusual for experts to disagree with findings of published articles. However, the ECT amnesia link as 'ridiculous', contradicting the fundamental basis of his own recent paper, is something else.

Another example of Hickie espousing diametrically opposing views is in relation to headspace. In his summary of research achievements of his four-million-dollar NHMRC Australia Fellowship, Hickie wrote in his final Fellowship report that his research had produced the evidence that headspace has produced 'substantial long-term improvements in functional outcomes':

The research associated with this Australia Fellowship set out, first, to implement and evaluate the effects of the new national youth mental health service network headspace and, second, to establish a discovery program for novel pathways to depression and anxiety. Not only have both aims been achieved but also the research and development enabled by this Australia Fellowship will help guarantee that headspace services thrive and provide integrated research platforms in the years to come. Outcomes to date, include the development of national and local mental health awareness designed to increase service utilisation as well as the provision of an evidence-base to help determine whether such new systems of targeted care result in substantial long-term improvements in functional outcomes. We now have the evidence to show that headspace has achieved this via the expansion and consolidation of both population-based and clinical aspects of mental health services.[482]

It is not clear when Hickie wrote this positive assessment of headspace. It was probably after 2012 (when his fellowship ended), and definitely before 13 June 2014, as the summary was included in an NHMRC compilation of grant reports with that cut-off date.[483]

Yet in April 2014, Hickie wrote a contradictory article, *Lack of headspace data a hindrance,* in which he was strongly critical of the lack of evidence about the effectiveness of headspace:

The range of services actually provided to young people is not clear. Importantly, whether these services are a real improvement on pre-existing service pathways has not yet been demonstrated... The emphasis on improving functional recovery through earlier intervention needs to be demonstrated.[484]

A few days later, the *Sydney Morning Herald* reported that Hickie was calling for an 'urgent, systematic national evaluation' of headspace, which he said had turned out to be 'high-cost, low-impact and low-population coverage'.

Extract from Bitter rift on youth mental health provider headspace

by Jill Stark in the *Sydney Morning Herald*, 13 April 2014.

A major rift within national youth mental health service headspace has erupted, with one of its founding board members publicly raising questions about how the organisation is run and whether it is reaching the vulnerable young people it was set up to help.

Ian Hickie, who was a key player in securing $420 million in early-intervention funding from the Gillard government, including the roll-out of 90 headspace drop-in centres across Australia, is now calling for an 'urgent, systematic national evaluation' of the organisation he helped build, claiming only half its centres are functional.

In a bitter feud which has seen lawyers engaged, headspace chief executive Chris Tanti described the claims as 'nonsense', saying they may be part of a backlash over the investigation of an incident at a Sydney headspace centre Professor Hickie runs through his Brain and Mind Research Institute, which remains in dispute.

However, this was rejected by Professor Hickie, one of Australia's most prominent psychiatrists. He acknowledged the 'confidential' review of clinical services was under way, but said his concerns were long-standing and shared by other major agencies in the mental health sector.

'It is worrying that Mr Tanti's assertions are an attempt once again to deflect public attention away from the open and appropriate reporting of the operations of headspace centres,' he said.

While Mr Tanti denied that half the centres were not functioning, he conceded after questioning from *The Sunday Age* that one in five were experiencing performance management issues related to workforce shortages, difficulties with external agencies, or low client numbers.

On average, each site saw 1000 young people a year, he said. 'Eighty per cent of our centres are functioning well and have good traction in their communities. A handful are not meeting performance requirements but are being actively managed. Most centres are seeing reasonable numbers of patients and have good uptake,' Mr Tanti said.

Professor Hickie first raised concerns in a keynote address at a youth mental health conference in February in Melbourne. He claimed the national rollout of headspace – the largest federal investment in the sector, intended to save money and lives by treating psychological distress early – had turned out to be 'high-cost, low-impact and low-population coverage'.[485]

This raises questions about Hickie's Australia Fellowship research. Does he stand by his claim in his Fellowship report that his research demonstrated that headspace has achieved 'substantial long-term improvements in functional outcomes'? If so, how can he reconcile this with his claims that headspace is 'high-cost, low-impact and low-population coverage' and that evidence about how *headspace* was performing was still lacking in 2014?

Which of Hickie's assessments should we believe? Given the four million dollars of tax-payers' money spent on Hickie's Australia Fellowship, the hundreds of millions of government funding for headspace, and headspace's central role in the delivery of mental health services for young Australians, this is more than just an academic issue.

Conflict with the *Lancet* editor over undeclared Conflicts of Interest

Hickie has played a major role in several depression awareness projects and antidepressant promotion activities funded by pharmaceutical companies.[486] This is not unusual for ambitious psychiatrists of his generation. Such links, when appropriately disclosed, do not constitute evidence of inappropriate relationships.

A noteworthy example of non-disclosure of an important conflict of interest occurred in May 2011, in an article published in *The Lancet,* one of the world's most prestigious medical journals. Hickie and Dr Naomi Rogers co-authored an evaluation of the use of melatonin analogues, commonly used to treat sleep disorders, for combating major depression.[487] The literature review extolled the virtues of agomelatine (brand name Valdoxan®), an antidepressant that is sold in the United Kingdom and Europe and Australia by French pharmaceutical company Servier.

Both Hickie and Rogers have significant financial links to Servier. Hickie was paid by Servier to do multiple presentations that promoted Valdoxan during 2010 and 2011. Although Rogers appropriately declared receiving honoraria for lectures from Servier, and Hickie declared some of his research ties to Servier, he did not declare his appearances at Valdoxan promotional events, either in the article or in the authors' response to criticism, published eight months later in *The Lancet.*

Hickie and Rogers' *Lancet* article strongly endorsed agomelatine. They claimed that agomelatine had advantages over other antidepressants, and they speculated that agomelatine 'might occupy a unique place in the management of some patients with severe depression and other major mood disorder'.[488]

Half of the abstract focused on the advantages of agomelatine. It prominently claimed that less than a quarter (23.9%) of patients taking agomelatine relapsed into depression, compared with half (50%) of patients who were given a placebo. However, that was only the case in one trial. The body of the paper, less likely to be read, admitted that 'two other relapse prevention trials did not indicate that agomelatine was more efficacious than placebo'.

The praise of agomelatine continued in the conclusion, which emphasised the superiority of agomelatine compared with other melatonin analogues: 'Importantly, only agomelatine… has been reported to have clinically significant antidepressant effects'.

Numerous researchers objected to the article. The January 2012 issue of *The Lancet* published six letters from researchers in America, Britain, France, Italy, and Australia, who were scathing in their criticism.[489] Among the problems identified were exaggeration of the efficacy of agomelatine, downplaying of potential harms, including liver toxicity, misrepresentation of the cited literature, and undeclared conflicts of interest.

A reply from Hickie and Rogers was published in the same issue.[490] Many of the detailed criticisms in the six letters, most notably the negative studies that were ignored, and the claims of misleadingly cited research were not addressed, in Hickie and Roger's reply.

The Lancet's Editor, Dr Richard Horton, was very critical of the review and acknowledged the shortcomings of *The Lancet*'s editorial process. The day before the six letters and the authors' reply was published, Horton began a series of tweets which stated:

> Tomorrow, we are very heavily criticised for publishing a review on melatonin-based drugs for depression. Biased and overstated, say many… The bias in this paper is very disturbing – it might be fine to argue your case in a Viewpoint or letter. But… this paper purported to be an unbiased review of a new drug class. Peer review improved it, yet not enough… As troubling is the fact that one author took part in speaking engagements for the company making one of these drugs… It is this kind of complicity that damages any hopes of a positive partnership between medicine and industry.[491]

Hickie was outraged and responded aggressively, claiming he had been defamed and demanded a retraction of Horton's public comments. in a *Crikey* article Hickie wrote:

> The content of the tweet is, in my view, clearly defamatory... I have lodged a complaint with the Ombudsman of *The Lancet* with a view to seeking a full retraction of the editor's defamatory public statements.[492]

Hickie's *Crikey* article went onto slam Horton and *The Lancet*:

> Horton has always been a controversial editor... In recent times, he has become a real celebrity in the UK, due largely to the edgy nature of his tweeting... To me *The Lancet*'s behaviour is considerably more commercial. In academe, as elsewhere, old-world publishers are rapidly losing the battle to free, online and open media outlets. Elsevier, the publishing house that produces *The Lancet*, is currently the subject of a worldwide boycott by some academics who are seeking a more open and transparent approach to the publication of science. In my view, *The Lancet*, through the agency of Horton's devotion to new media, is desperate to attract wider public attention before it goes out of business. From an armchair in central London, causing harm to individual academics, or a process like mental health reform in Australia, is a very minor concern.[493]

Hickie's *Crikey* article did not address the substantive criticisms of his and Roger's paper – exaggeration of the efficacy and downplaying the risks of agomelatine. He described these concerns as 'unfounded', without elaborating. Instead, his *Crikey* article concentrated on the details of his capacity to declare promotional activities for Servier that he claimed he was unable to declare:

> Given that we... started returning proof corrections in February

2011, it was not possible to declare key educational or media activities supporter [sic] by Servier that occurred later in 2011.[494]

However, Hickie had done at least one promotional event for Servier well before February 2011 that he did not declare in the original article. He presented at a Servier Foundation Depression Masterclass on 5 November 2010,[495] three months before he started returning proof corrections in February 2011. He also presented at Servier Valdoxan masterclasses on 19 February and 5 March 2011. Then he was the main presenter at a Servier briefing on 11 April and was fulsome in his praise for Valdoxan in media coverage of the event.[496] This was still more than one month before publication of the early online version of the article on 18 May 2011.

His partner, Elizabeth Scott, was also a paid presenter at the 19 February 2011 Valdoxan masterclass and the 11 April 2011 briefing, but she failed to declare this in a paper submitted to *Translational Psychiatry* on 6 December 2011.[497] She eventually disclosed her honoraria in a corrigendum in 2013[498], after Melissa Raven contacted the journal publisher's head office after having been repeatedly ignored by the editor of *Translational Psychiatry*.

Hickie got it wrong when he failed to declare the Servier Valdoxan marketing payments in his and Rogers' original article. He got it wrong again later in their reply to critics in *The Lancet*, when he asserted that his 'financial relationships with Servier Laboratories (and other government and industry-related entities) were disclosed exhaustively at the time of publication'[499] He then tripled down on his error in his *Crickey* article when he again wrongly claimed he had 'clearly stated them all at the end of the original article' and that his critics were defaming him.[500] For obvious reasons Hickie never got the retraction he demanded from Horton.

While this does not inspire confidence in Professor Hickie, I believe the initial omission was a relatively minor problem. A busy clinician/researcher/entrepreneur with extensive financial ties to the pharmaceutical industry could easily forget to declare one source of payments. It is an understandable and forgivable error. A bigger issue is that Hickie and Rogers failed to address substantive criticisms of biased methods and findings, either in their authors' reply in *The Lancet*[501], or in Hickie's *Crikey* article.

When the *Lancet* controversy broke, Hickie was one of eight National Mental Health Commissioners tasked with providing 'expert and independent advice to the [Australian] Government on the performance of our mental health system'.[502] Because of his behaviour, I told *The Australian* newspaper that Hickie should 'step aside as a mental health commissioner', adding 'if he doesn't [Mental Health Minister] Mark Butler should remove him'.[503] However, Butler backed Hickie without addressing the substantive issues summarised by the Lancet editor. Eight years later, Hickie remains a very influential and a prominent media spokesperson, particularly on the ABC and in mainstream newspapers, in relation to mental health.

InnoWell: entrepreneurial e-mental health

A current example of Hickie's problematic potential conflicts of interest is the InnoWell initiative – a joint venture by PricewaterhouseCoopers (PwC) and the University of Sydney, with Hickie owning a 5% stake. Hickie has described InnoWell as 'a technology-enabled solution to reform mental health care services' that provides digital tools to enable health professionals to better understand how clients/patients are progressing.[504] According to PwC:

> InnoWell... aims to use technology to help medical professionals
> and health providers better connect with and monitor the
> people that use their services... the InnoWell Platform, which

provides medical professionals and health services with tools to better understand where the person using their service is at and track their progress. For health providers, it provides crucial information they can use to triage patients, ensuring those with the most immediate need are seen first. It also allows them to monitor the effectiveness of treatments and programs to aid their decision making for the future.[505]

In a 2019 article, *Making better choices about mental health investment: The case for urgent reform of Australia's Better Access Program*, Hickie and co-author Sebastian Rosenberg argued for 'an increased role for incorporation of digital technologies alongside clinical services' in the Better Access program, which they strongly criticised. One of their specific recommendations was to 'incentivise the adoption of digitally supported psychological services'.

You might think that, after the *Lancet* controversy, Hickie would have taken extra care with his conflict of interest declarations. However, the Declaration of Conflicting Interests did not mention Hickie's stake in InnoWell, instead stating: 'The author(s) declared no potential conflicts of interest with respect to the research, authorship, and/or publication of this article'.[506]

Similarly, there is no mention of Hickie's stake in InnoWell in a recent Brain and Mind Centre publication, *Rethinking Mental Health in Australia*, that he co-authored, that explicitly aims to influence government policy and promotes digital solutions similar to those provided by InnoWell.[507]

In summary, Ian Hickie is a mental health entrepreneur. There is nothing inherently wrong with that. We need mental health innovators, and salesmanship is an essential part of entrepreneurship. But entrepreneurs are not neutral, independent experts, and salesmanship is not science. It is inappropriate for the government and media to treat Hickie as an unbiased commentator or advisor, and inappropriate for the media to quote him without disclosing his potential conflicts of interest. Hickie is a player, not an impartial umpire.

I believe that, more than any other individual, Hickie has played a lead role in driving Australia's soaring rates of depression diagnosis and antidepressant use. He has persuasively promoted the message that depression is massively under-recognised and under-treated, and many of us have bought it.

Chapter 8

Australia's BioPsychiatry Channel (the ABC)

A particularly disappointing aspect of our national debate on mental health has been our national broadcaster's uncritical promotion of Professors McGorry and Hickie as authoritative, independent, trustworthy mental health gurus.

One example was ABC radio's *The World Today*'s coverage of the Hickie-*Lancet* controversy. The coverage was troubling, mostly for what it omitted. Adelaide psychiatrist, Professor Jon Jureidini, who was one of the 11 authors highly critical of Hickie's paper, is quoted in the transcript of *The World Today*: 'The authors had financial and other relationships with the manufacturer of the drug… There are concerns about the misrepresentation of the effectiveness of the drug, about the clinical usefulness of it, about its adverse effects and about conflicts of interest.'

Hickie responded to Jureidini's criticisms, saying they were 'a slur on us, it's a slur on the journal [*The Lancet*] and its editorial processes'. Hickie's close colleague, Adjunct Professor John Mendoza, defended Hickie, saying 'Ian is very mindful of these things. I mean you don't get asked to write pieces for *The Lancet* unless you have a high standing in terms of your scientific rigor and approach.'[508]

The ABC and Mendoza missed the main point of the story. It made no reference to the fact that it was the Editor of *The Lancet*,

Richard Horton, who was Hickie's most strident critic. Horton also acknowledged and accepted the criticisms of *The Lancet*'s publication policies and identified changes to improve them. *The World Today*'s coverage mentioned none of this. Instead, readers and listeners were left with the impression that *The Lancet* and Hickie were on the same side of the argument. The *World Today* program and Hickie's implied defence of the integrity of *The Lancet* aired on 13 February 2012. Two days later, Hickie's *Crikey* article, containing his damming assessment of *The Lancet* and its Editor, Horton – including Hickie's claim that Horton had defamed him – was published (see Chapter 7).[509] As he had with ECT-induced amnesia and headspace (see Chapter 7), Hickie demonstrated his capacity to expound two contradictory views – in this case, simultaneously!

The final comment in the *World Today* program (titled 'Psychiatrist claims campaign to discredit him') was left to Mendoza, who said it was a 'vicious personal campaign' against Hickie by people who Mendoza bizarrely claimed 'still want to hold onto old 19th century-style institutional beds'. Neither Hickie nor Mendoza, nor the ABC, addressed any of the substantive issues raised. Instead, the article ended with Mendoza defending Hickie from conflict of interest criticisms by arguing that Hickie drove inexpensive cars and lived in a humble home.[510]

At the time, Hickie was a National Mental Health Commissioner whose advice was relied upon by the Australian Government to 'provide expert and independent advice to the Government on the performance of our mental health system'. Professor Hickie was the only psychiatrist on the Commission, This story should have been a big deal – a senior expert advisor to government had been criticised for 'cash for comment' type behaviour by the editor of one of the world's most prestigious journals. But the ABC's coverage left the impression that a bunch of disgruntled rivals were taking on Professor Hickie and *The Lancet*.

In the case of Professor McGorry, the ABC seems unduly impressed by the fact that he is a former Australian of the Year. One notable example of the ABC's promotion of McGorry was when, in 2014, driven by the then Managing Director Mark Scott, the ABC ran a Telethon style event that raised 'more than $1 million' for research driven by McGorry.[511] The Telethon was the final event in a week-long *Mental As* campaign to raise awareness and funds for mental health research. The genesis was a meeting between Scott and McGorry.[512] The ABC 'worked closely' with the pharmaceutical industry funded *Mental Health Australia*[513] in developing the campaign.

Most of the *Mental As* coverage was uncontroversial and encouraged good mental health habits. However, there was a consistent theme of massive unmet need, and promises of safe, effective treatments, including medications, if only troubled Australians sought professional help. The coverage concluded with a chorus of circular praise between McGorry, Scott and the ABC.

The most disturbing element of the *Mental As* coverage was not what the ABC showed, but what was deliberately excluded. The ABC had commissioned a one-hour documentary to be produced by then ABC journalist, Dr Maryanne Demasi as part of the *Mental As* week coverage. She worked in the science unit of the ABC as an experienced TV journalist who was a former medical researcher.

I was approached by Demasi in relation to the concerns I had expressed in the Western Australian Parliament about McGorry and Hickie endorsing the use of antidepressants as a means of preventing youth suicide.[514] The documentary was going to shine a light on the link between antidepressants and youth suicide (detailed in chapter 4) and would feature influential psychiatrists like Hickie and McGorry who seemed to think there was evidence for their use in people under the age of 18. Demasi has subsequently advised me that Hickie and McGorry were going to be interviewed but they were very unhappy that their critics – including Australian Professor of Psychiatry Jon Jureidini, UK Professor of Psychiatry David Healy and Danish physician Professor Peter Gøtzsche – were also being interviewed.

Demasi advised me that the ABC management tried to appease Hickie and McGorry by demanding that she delete bits of commentary that were critical of them, but Demasi refused. Apparently management suggested that Demasi dump Gøtzsche's interview entirely from the documentary, because they feared that his views were too controversial. Eventually, Hickie and McGorry declined to be a part of the documentary.

Demasi told me that the ABC management decided that, without McGorry and Hickie's input, the documentary would lack 'balance' and that ABC Managing Director Mark Scott ordered it to be killed off, only weeks before it was due to air. Demasi's account is consistent with the account of Professor Peter Gøtzsche outlined in his book *Deadly Psychiatry and Organised Denial.*[515]

In April 2015, not long after ABC management killed Demasi's story, the ABC's *7.30 Report* obtained a leaked copy of the *National Mental Health Commission* report[516] into Australia's mental health system. The Commission's report stated that the current system was poorly planned and integrated and was a 'massive drain on people's wellbeing'. It urged a 'radical rethink of responses' to mentally ill people seeking help and recommended redirecting more than $1 billion in funding from acute hospital care to community-based mental health services.

Professors McGorry and Mendoza were the only two mental health experts interviewed by *7.30*. Mendoza spoke about a recent family tragedy. His nephew, Jeff Mendoza, was one of two examples referred to of young men suiciding after being turned out of acute mental health services prematurely and without adequate support.

Excerpt from Transcript of ABC's *7.30 Report* April 2015[517]

JOHN MENDOZA, FMR MENTAL HEALTH CHIEF ADVISER: I was driving at the time when my brother rang me and it was a call I'll never forget.

SABRA LANE (ABC Journalist): Last November, Jeff Mendoza warned his family he was planning to kill himself. Frantic, they called police who put Jeff under an emergency examination order and took him to the Gold Coast University Hospital for an urgent mental health assessment. Yet he was discharged the next day.

DI MENDOZA: No one can even tell me how he left the hospital. I know that they discharged him. I know they gave him a script – this is a script. He had no wallet. He had no shoes. He was dressed in a hospital gown. I don't even know how he got home.

JOHN MENDOZA: I know that what service Jeff was afforded when the police brought him to the Gold Coast University Hospital was, frankly, appalling. And a dog hit by a car gets a better standard of care than what he did. And I have no doubt today that if he was afforded better care on that occasion, back in November last year, he'd be here today.

SABRA LANE: Within 30 hours of leaving hospital, Jeff killed himself.

JOHN MENDOZA: There was, you know, a plan to give him a phone call on the Saturday – which they did. They actually rang an hour after he had died.

SABRA LANE: For Professor Mendoza, Jeff's death has painfully brought home what he's known for years: the mental health system is a mish-mash of shared responsibilities between State, Federal and local bodies.

JOHN MENDOZA: We have a shemozzle and the shemozzle has to end because it is costing lives. It's costing our nation dearly.

SABRA LANE: In opposition, the Coalition made a review of mental health services a priority and ordered it when it won Government. It was conducted by the National Mental Health Commission. Its report was handed to the Government last November.

It hasn't been made public but *7.30* has obtained key parts of it. The commission says there's an overwhelming case for a 'radical rethink of responses' to mentally ill people seeking help. It says the system's poorly planned and integrated and is a 'massive drain on people's wellbeing'. It finds 'major deficiencies in the response received by many of those seeking help for suicidal thinking, attempts or bereavement'. The report says there is substantial funding within the mental health system but that it's not distributed efficiently, effectively or fairly.

It makes the significant recommendation that, from 2017, the Federal Government redirect more than $1 billion earmarked for acute hospital care and pump it into community-based mental health services instead.

JOHN MENDOZA: We are still spending more than 50% of our mental health funding in acute care hospital wards. Wrong. The evidence to support that does not exist. What we should be doing is shifting that funding to the community sector. We should be ensuring that we have the capacity to reach out to people like Jeffrey in crisis, treat them in their home.

SABRA LANE: Professor Mendoza quit his position as chief adviser on mental health to the Rudd government in 2010 over its inaction and he says it's time for this Government to prove it's serious about reform.

JOHN MENDOZA: So in 2010, 2011 again, Tony Abbott made mental health matter. Now was that merely political opportunism? Or was the Prime Minister genuine in terms of a commitment to mental health reform? I don't know the answer to that. But the longer this report is not released, the more it looks like opportunism.

SABRA LANE: A former Australian of the Year and mental health expert, Patrick McGorry believes Australia is at a crossroads and he says he has faith the Government is committed to releasing the review.

PATRICK MCGORRY, EXEC. DIR., ORYGEN YOUTH MENTAL HEALTH: Well, the first thing is to make the public aware of what a preventable killer it actually is. And then we need evidence-based strategies to stem the tide and set targets and reduction of suicide. For example, in Sweden they set a zero road toll target by 2020. We should at least set a 50% reduction target in suicide over the next five to 10 years.

SABRA LANE: The review finds more people die by their own hand than are killed in road accidents or skin cancer and it notes, while Australia's road toll has more than halved in 40 years, there's been little change in the suicide rate. Two thousand, five hundred and thirty-five people were killed in 2012: double the road toll.

PATRICK MCGORRY: Well, with the suicide figures as shocking as they are and the suicide attempts at this almost epidemic rate, the reason the public are not demanding action is because they're not aware of these facts, not sufficiently aware of those facts.

The ABC's coverage raised some very important issues. It highlighted that the system is a 'mish-mash of shared responsibilities between State, Federal and local bodies' and 'the system is so broken that it often hurts the people it's supposed to help'. It also identified the need for more support in the community. All of these criticisms are valid; however, again the ABC's coverage was problematic because of what was left out, rather than what was included.

The fact that the key recommendation of the report was to strip $1 billion out of acute hospital care, the system that turned away Mendoza's nephew and the other young man, seems to have been completely lost on both Mendoza and the ABC reporters. Yes, more money is needed for community care, and too often acute services harm more than they help, but is stripping them of $1 billion really going to improve outcomes? The possibility that antidepressant use may have contributed to the suicide of these young men was also completely ignored. Also ignored was the possibility that, by funding headspace and EPPIC services – as demanded by McGorry, Hickie and Mendoza – the Commonwealth Government had contributed to the fragmentation of the system referred to in the coverage.

McGorry's call for 'evidence-based strategies to stem the tide' and for government to set a national target of a 50% drop in suicides in the 'next 5 to 10 years', was particularly galling. The possibility that McGorry's and Hickie's dismissal of the FDA warning had contributed to rising youth suicide rates was going to be a theme of the story Demasi was prevented from preparing by ABC management. Yet, a few months later, McGorry on the ABC was again being portrayed as the expert with the capacity to save lives.

More recently, in June 2019, *7.30* presented a piece – *Managing the maze of child mental health*[518] – about the risks and benefits for children and teenagers of using antidepressants. It told the story of two teenage boys and their families. One boy, Eden, aged 13, had been 'medicated' with antidepressants for five years, and the other, Henry, aged 12, had not. Both were presented as success stories that illustrated how different pathways can have their challenges but can be successful.

Eden was eight when he was diagnosed with anxiety. At 12, he was also diagnosed with depression. He had also previously been diagnosed with autism spectrum disorder. Eden had attempted suicide and self-harmed, and had been violent with his mother and other students after he was medicated. The story made no mention of the fact that no antidepressant is approved for use by children (under 18) in Australia. Even more importantly, it made no mention of the FDA or TGA suicidality warnings. I wrote to the journalist, Andy Park, asking him if Eden's parents, Jodie and John had been made aware of the suicidality risk. I got no response, and subsequently I complained to the ABC and sent the information to the ABC's *Media Watch* program. Again there was no response.

The best that we can hope about Andy Park's editorial comment that 'prescriptions… have been successful as in Eden's case' was that he was ignorant of the FDA suicidality warning. If Park or anyone at the ABC's *7.30* editorial team knew of the warning and didn't cover it in the story (particularly given Eden's history of suicidality and self-harm), this was biased journalism. If they didn't know about the warning, it was ignorant journalism. Either way it was bad journalism.

Australia needs a vigorous national debate about the future of mental health, but our taxpayer funded national broadcaster is at best ignorant of significant facts, and at worst is stifling debate and promoting the unchallenged views of a few gurus. McGorry and Hickie deserve credit for putting mental health on the national political agenda, and many of their criticisms of the current system are indisputable. However, just because you can point at a problem doesn't mean you know the solution; and if you are paid to promote pharmaceuticals, you are not independent.

After a decade of McGorry and Hickie having substantial influence over the direction of national mental health policy, the ABC needs to begin to hold them to account. When the ABC picks favourites and ignores contradictory evidence, our national debate dumbs down. Other contradictory voices need to be heard on 'our' ABC.

We need an ABC that elevates debate and deals with big issues without fear or favour. The future of Australia's mental health system is a crucial and complex issue. Millions of Australians, either directly, or indirectly as family and friends, have the potential to be either helped or harmed. It requires better coverage than the black and white bumper sticker campaign that has been run at the ABC for the last decade. The slow death of viable private sector investigative journalism caused by plummeting newspaper revenue streams makes the ABC even more important. We need a critical media interested in robust evidence. We certainly don't need a crusading taxpayer funded national broadcaster that lacks objectivity, picks a side, and sticks with it by ignoring contradictory evidence.

Chapter 9

The TGA: Australia's Soft Touch Regulator

One of the positives to come out of COVID19 is an increase in political, media and public interest in health policy and the operations of Australia's medical product safety regulator the Therapeutic Goods Administration (TGA). As discussed at the end of Chapter 4, there is some reason to be hopeful that the TGA may be upping its performance at least in regard to the post-market analysis of the safety of antidepressants. However, there is massive room for improvement.

A first priority should be reforming the TGA's product licencing processes. Typically, they involve drug or medical device manufacturers providing cherry-picked favourable evidence to the TGA, which uses this biased evidence to assess the product's approval for a specific purpose (an on-label use). Once the product is licenced, doctors are generally free to prescribe it as they judge fit, even if it is not approved for this purpose (off label use).

The TGA often never sees unfavourable evidence before drugs are approved for market. The product manufacturers have total discretion in what information they provide to the TGA. Even if product manufacturers were compelled to provide all the research they conducted to the TGA, this might not improve matters much. By carefully choosing and rewarding those who do the research that provides the evidence about their products, they can virtually guarantee a favourable evidence base.

Furthermore, because drug companies are regarded as legal 'persons', the documents they provide to the Commonwealth Government health regulators and agencies have the same exemption as patient records from Freedom of Information (FOI) requirements under section 135A of the National Health Act 1953.[519] The Health Act was written to protect patient privacy; but now perversely helps to hide the details of how Big Pharma influences the TGA. So, despite the fact that it is our taxes that subsidise many of these drugs through the PBS, and it is our bodies that ingest the drugs, we are not allowed see the safety and efficacy evidence used to persuade our government to licence and subsidise drugs.

How I inadvertently helped Big Pharma hide safety and efficacy data

In 2010, a Freedom of Information case adjudicated by the Administrative Appeals Tribunal (Whitely and Department of Health and Ageing [2010] AATA 338) established a legal precedent that prevents public scrutiny of documents provided by corporations to the Commonwealth Department of Health and Ageing (DoHA).[520] [521]

I was the unsuccessful plaintiff in the case. Citing public interest provisions of Commonwealth Freedom of Information legislation, I requested copies of all safety and efficacy data provided to DoHA by drug company Eli Lily supporting its application to get the ADHD drug Strattera (atomoxetine hydrochloride) subsidised via the Pharmaceutical Benefits Scheme (PBS). I wanted to understand why the DoHA had decided it was in the public interest to subsidise an ADHD drug that carried a black box warning for suicide and a second warning for potentially fatal liver damage (and later a third for cardiovascular damage).

DoHA had originally recognised 11 documents as being relevant. Eli Lily opposed the release of eight of these documents to me. The DoHA decided to release two documents in full, and provided me with heavily redacted (virtually unreadable) copies of seven documents. I was denied access to the two other documents. I appealed this decision, and asked for access to all documents, with appropriate redactions for commercially sensitive information about production costs and pricing. (I was only interested in safety and efficacy data.)

The Administrative Appeals Tribunal was convinced by lawyers acting for Eli Lily and DoHA that, for the purpose of the National Health Act (1953), all corporations are 'persons', and therefore under Section 38(1) of the Australian FOI Act and Section 135A(1) of the Health Act 1953, their documents have the same privacy protections as a patient's medical records (and were therefore exempt from FOI requests).

Section 135A(1) states:

> A person shall not, directly or indirectly, except in the performance of duties, or in the exercise of powers or functions, under this Act or for the purpose of enabling a person to perform functions under the Medicare Australia Act 1973 or the medical indemnity legislation, and while the person is, or after the person ceases to be, an officer, divulge or communicate to any person, any information with respect to the affairs of a third person acquired by the first-mentioned person in the performance of duties, or in the exercise of powers or functions, under this Act. Penalty: $5,000 or imprisonment for 2 years, or both.

My appeal was a spectacular failure. I lost the ability to publicise disturbing elements of the documents I already had. Worse still, it created a precedent that prevents public scrutiny of drug safety documents that we should have access to.

This law works really well for Big Pharma, but not for consumers. Once a dodgy product is approved for market, it is almost impossible to get the information required to get it taken off market. The TGA onus of proof is effectively reversed, so that consumers damaged by unsafe drugs and medical devices have to prove beyond any doubt that the products are unfit for market.

This is where we have been for the last 15 years in regards to the relationship between antidepressant use and youth suicide. As discussed in Chapter 4, in August 2005 the TGA responded half-heartedly to the FDA's black box warning by deciding not to issue the equivalent boxed warning, but instead required the rewording of Product Information and Consumer Information leaflets made available to doctors and consumers.[522] The TGA's limp response was typical of its approach at the time. From January to September 2005, the FDA issued twenty black box warnings for prescription drugs that were sold in both the US and Australia, but the TGA issued equivalent warnings for only five of them.[523]

The default response of the TGA has been that it accepts that products are safe unless it can be shown beyond doubt that a product is extremely harmful. Occasionally, there are spectacular regulatory failures causing hundreds of deaths or destroying lives that become so obvious that even the regulator, has to admit it erred (e.g. Vioxx[524], Pradaxa[525], metal hips[526], transvaginal mesh[527] and PIP breast implants[528]).

Vioxx and Pradaxa's trails of death

In 2004, after causing an estimated 60,000 deaths worldwide primarily from heart attacks and strokes, Merck pharmaceutical's bestselling arthritis drug Vioxx was withdrawn from sale worldwide. Prior to that, Merck had 'mounted a ghost-writing campaign' to promote Vioxx. Ninety-six articles were published, some of which omitted to mention the deaths of patients who participated in clinical trials of the drug.[529] Not only did it promote dishonest conduct, Merck had 'drawn up a hit list of "rogue" researchers who had criticised Vioxx [who] had to be discredited and 'neutralized'.[530] [531]

Vioxx is not an isolated example of a drug company concealing evidence relating to the safety of one of their drugs. More recently (in 2014) it was revealed that Boehringer Ingelheim, the maker of anti-coagulant drug Pradaxa, had withheld some of their internal analysis that suggested that patients should have their blood levels monitored. A *BMJ* investigation found that Boehringer Ingelheim did not release the analysis because it did not fit in with its marketing strategy.[532] Pradaxa had been heavily marketed as a drug that did not require patients to monitor blood levels, as opposed to the market leading anti-coagulant Warfarin.

Pradaxa has been 'associated with 280 deaths in Australia and 1,400 adverse drug reactions in the past five years, including abdominal bleeding, brain haemorrhages, strokes and heart attacks.' [533] This compared to Warfarin, which has been linked 'to 30 deaths and 270 reactions over the same period.' [534] Boehringer Ingelheim disputes that they ever withheld relevant data from regulators, despite the fact that they are paying out $650 million to settle 4,000 lawsuits across the United States.[535]

Boehringer Ingelheim's internal research by one of its own clinical program directors, Dr Paul A. Reilly, had shown that there was an 'optimal plasma concentration' which could be attained through blood monitoring and which would be beneficial for some patients.[536] An internal email from a company supervisor stated that she could not believe that this research might be published by the company, an act that would undermine a decade's worth of work. She further added that it would be 'extremely difficult' to defend to the regulating authorities the company's claim that blood monitoring was not needed. 'I would like to ask you to check again whether this is really wanted,' she wrote about publishing the research.[537] Another internal email, by yet another company official, stated that 'the publication [of the article] will [do] more harm than be useful for us… but especially harmful in the discussions with regulatory bodies'.[538]

When the research paper by Dr Reilly was published in the *Journal of the American College of Cardiology*, the research indicating that there was an optimal blood-level range had been omitted.[539] This information only came to light when an Illinois judge who was overseeing thousands of lawsuits lodged by people who claimed that Boehringer Ingleheim did not properly warn them about the risks of taking Pradaxa released drug company documents.[540]

Boehringer Ingleheim ended up settling the Pradaxa lawsuits in 2014 for over US$650 million.[541] Enormous fines and settlement payments like that for Pradaxa seem to be accepted as just part of the cost of doing business for many of the world's largest pharmaceutical companies. From 2004 to 2013 in the USA, at least $19.47 billion in fines and settlements were paid for off-label promotion and marketing and fraudulent misbranding and marketing.[542] Companies fined include Johnson & Johnson, GlaxoSmithKline, Abbott, Novartis, Forest, AstraZeneca, Pfizer, Eli Lilly, Bristol-Myers Squibb, and Purdue.

The latest high-profile drug scandal that Australians are yet to fully comprehend is the misuse of pharmaceutical opioids. In the USA, the opioid crisis has claimed a staggering 400,000 lives over the past two decades.[543] This scandal has received enough publicity in Australia to sound warning bells. However, there is little evidence of an appropriate response so far.

Excerpt from Opioid crisis goes global as deaths surge in Australia
AP News 6 September 2019 [544]

… Half a world away, Australia has failed to heed the lessons of the United States, and is now facing skyrocketing rates of opioid prescriptions and related deaths. Drug companies facing scrutiny for their aggressive marketing of opioids in America have turned their focus abroad, working around marketing regulations to push the painkillers in other countries. And as with the U.S., Australia's government has also been slow to respond to years of warnings from worried health experts...

Australia's death rate from opioids has more than doubled in just over a decade. And health experts worry that without urgent action, Australia is on track for an even steeper spike in deaths like those seen in America, where the epidemic has left 400,000 dead...

More than 3 million Australians – an eighth of the country's population – are getting at least one opioid prescription a year, according to the latest data...

In Australia, pharmaceutical companies by law cannot directly advertise to consumers, but are free to market the drugs to medical professionals. And they have done so, aggressively and effectively, by sponsoring swanky conferences, running doctors' training seminars, funding research papers, giving money to pain advocacy groups and meeting with doctors to push the drugs for chronic pain...

David Tonkin blames his son's death on a system that allowed him to see 24 doctors and get 23 different medications from 16 pharmacies – all in the space of six months. Between January and July 2014 alone, Matthew Tonkin got 27 prescriptions just for oxycodone.

Matthew Tonkin's tragic death, like so many others prescription drug overdose deaths, was predictable and avoidable. For well over a decade, many prominent voices, including state coroners, prominent pharmacists and the Australian Medical Association, have called for the nationwide roll-out of real time monitoring of the dispensing of frequently abused prescription drugs. In May 2011, I told the Western Australian Minister for Health, Kim Hames, in the WA State Parliament:

> It may take some cooperation between state and federal governments, but all that needs to happen is for pharmacists' computers to be able to talk to each other so that when somebody has a script filled faster than it could possibly be used, assuming that there are adequate identification processes in place, it can be identified that the person should not be prescribed further drugs to avoid potential abuse. It is a really simple solution to a really big and growing problem, and it would not be particularly expensive to implement. There may be some privacy implications that need to be considered, but we simply need computer networks that can talk to each other, and that is surely not beyond our wit and wisdom to get [state and federal governments] together and solve this problem. (See Appendix 1.)

I was obviously wrong. Despite 15 years of repeated calls from coroners, pharmacists groups, the Australian Medical Association, and numerous false starts, it has proved way beyond the wit and wisdom of our state and federal leaders to implement a system that will save lives and money.

Most regulatory failures are less clear-cut than those for Vioxx, Pradaxa and OxyContin. More often, the TGA extends a considerable benefit of doubt to product manufacturers, as they have done for ADHD drug Strattera.

Straterra's Sad Story

Atomoxetine Hydrochloride (brand name Strattera) is a noradrenaline reuptake inhibitor. It was first trialled in the 1980s as an antidepressant branded Tomoxetine but was found to be ineffective.[545] It was licensed in the USA in 2002 for the treatment of ADHD, particularly in patients who don't get a therapeutic response or who experience side effects from stimulant medication. Unlike stimulants, atomoxetine is not considered addictive and is not diverted for illicit use, but does not have immediate effects and can take up to six weeks before it modifies ADHD behavioural symptoms.[546]

Strattera came onto the Australian market in early 2004. It was licensed by the TGA on the back of evidence from two studies chosen by its manufacturer, Eli Lilly. Elli Lilly chose who conducted the studies and had the opportunity to 'cherry pick' favourable studies (and ignore unfavourable studies) to support its' licensing application.

Despite claims of Strattera being a milder ADHD drug, concerns soon emerged about its safety. On 17 December 2004, the US FDA issued a talk paper, 'New Warning for Strattera', which stated:

> The drug's labeling is being updated with a bolded warning about the potential for severe liver injury in patients taking Strattera. The label warns that severe liver injury can progress to liver failure in a small percentage of patients. It cautions clinicians to discontinue the drug in patients who develop jaundice or laboratory evidence of liver injury. It also notes that the actual number of cases of severe liver injury from the drug is not known because of under-reporting.[547]

Less than a year later, on 29 September 2005, the FDA issued a public health advisory, announcing they had put the highest possible black box warning on Strattera for suicidal ideation:

> Strattera increases the risk of suicidal thinking in children and adolescents with ADHD. Patients who are started on therapy should be observed closely for clinical worsening, suicidal thinking or behaviours, or unusual changes in behaviour. Families and caregivers should be advised to closely observe the patient and to communicate changes or concerning behaviours with the prescriber.[548]

In March 2006, the TGA followed the FDA's lead and issued an equivalent 'suicidality' warning to prescribers. However, unlike the FDA, the TGA made no attempt to alert the media or the public and left that responsibility to individual doctors.

In November 2011, the TGA added a warning about 'clinically significant increases in heart rate and blood pressure'.[549] The safety advisory warns:

> Atomoxetine [Strattera] is contraindicated in patients with symptomatic cardiovascular diseases, moderate to severe hypertension or severe cardiovascular disorders, whose condition would be expected to deteriorate if they experienced increases in blood pressure or in heart rate that could be clinically important.

There have been numerous reports of severe adverse events, including completed suicides by children taking Strattera. However, because many adverse events are not reported to regulatory authorities the prevalence of these effects is not known.[550]

A Sample from the Adverse Drug Reactions Committee (ADRAC) adverse event reports for Atomoxetine Hydrochloride (Strattera)[551]

- 8 year old boy who 'hit his head against a wall' and had 'thoughts of suicide – stating that he wants to kill himself'

- 12 year old girl who experienced; 'anorexia, weight loss, fidgeting and compulsive behaviour that included ripping out fingernails and toenails, picking and cutting clothing, and anger outbursts'

- 7 year old girl who 'became very agitated while travelling in the family car and had explosive mood swings. She said that she intended to open the door and get out of the car, and she tried to open the car door'

- 9 year old boy who 'developed abnormal behaviour, including strange facial expressions with bilateral eyelid ptosis and became very emotionally withdrawn'

- 9 year old boy who displayed 'aggression, was totally irrational for three days and became violent, all of which was totally out of character'

- 13 year old boy who 'experienced chest pains and hostile and aggressive behaviour, but the problems immediately disappeared with the cessation of Strattera'

- 9 year old boy who slammed 'his head against walls, had extreme mood swings, violent outbursts' and was 'always angry, depressed or sad and said he wanted to kill himself'

- 10 year old boy who 'experienced nausea, then became acutely depressed, aggressive and had suicidal thoughts'

- 7 year old girl who experienced 'abdominal pain, nausea, severe right sided headache, shooting pains, white spots in visual fields, academic regression and faecal and urinary incontinence'

- 7 year old boy who experienced 'suicidal ideation and mood changes' and suffered from 'increased aggression' and 'threats to self with knife, picking his skin, poking self with knife'

- 12 year old boy experienced 'very strong suicidal ideation… talking about dead bodies and about hanging himself'

- 11 year old boy who 'attempted suicide' and who experienced 'headache(s), stomach cramps, muscle rigidity and poor concentration'

- 7 year old boy who experienced 'suicidal ideation'

- 10 year old boy who developed 'psychotic symptoms' and began 'talking about suicide'

- 11 year old boy who experienced 'a psychotic episode and took an overdose of his mother's thyroxine'

- 9 year old boy who 'experienced suicidal thoughts'

- 11 year old boy who became 'extremely agitated' and 'talked about wanting to die'

- 13 year old boy who experienced 'suicidal ideation, physical and verbal aggression to family' and became 'angry, withdrawn, socially isolatory, impulsive, moody'

- 11 year old boy who 'took Strattera for the treatment of ADHD to complement Ritalin, under the influence of which he became suicidal and depressed'

- 12 year old girl who 'ripped out her fingernails and toenails'

- 9 year old girl who 'experienced self-harming'

- 9 year old boy who expressed 'suicidal ideation', 'aggression' and 'self-harm' and made 'drawings of him hanging upside down from a tree, in (the) ocean'

- 10 year old boy who was psychotic and experienced auditory hallucinations including 'hearing voices in his head to kill his sister'

- 15 year old girl who experienced suicidal ideation and started cutting herself to the extent that was 'life threatening'

- 14 year old girl who 'started cutting herself. It was reported that she felt compelled to start cutting herself and cut her arms with razors, scissors, knives. The patient had suicidal ideation while causing self-harm'

- 8 year old boy who was 'talking about killing himself/suicide. Patient was not depressed and discussed suicide in a boastful manner. Treating paediatrician continued atomoxetine and considered adding Risperidone. Past history included sexual abuse'

- 10 year old boy who had 'suicidal thoughts and threats, despair/depression... and violent outbursts'

- and a 13 year old boy who 'commenced on Strattera ... and was more agitated than usual and extremely strong suicidal ideation and urges – he climbed on a roof to jump off. Also had extremely strong ideation to seriously hurt and put in intensive care some of the other schoolchildren.'

Note: On 1 October 2013, after the suicide of a 9-year-old boy, the TGA restated its suicide warning for Strattera.[552]

In 2012, the TGA stopped making individual de-identified adverse event reports available on request. They justified the decision on privacy grounds. However, it is difficult to see how any individual could be identified, out of population of more than 25 million, from information like that detailed above. Instead, the TGA now provides intermittent summaries of adverse events on their website.

The TGA's industry friendly approach is reinforced by the fact that, in Australia, adverse event reporting for drugs and medical devices is voluntary. As a result, only a fraction of incidents are reported to the TGA.[553] This leads to an unrealistically favourable perception of the safety of many drugs and devices that is rarely, if ever, challenged by the TGA. If there was full public access to all the relevant safety data and compulsory adverse event reporting, we would have a true picture of the real risks and benefits of drugs like Strattera. Many drugs that are currently assumed to be safe and effective may be shown to be anything but.

Australia needs a robust, independent, evidence-based regulator that has the power and resources, and most importantly the will, to intervene to protect consumer safety. Despite some recent encouraging steps, there is a long way to go before that is the case.

Chapter 10

Where to from here?

In the not-too-distant past, extremely damaging, life-destroying or life-ending psychiatric practices, like lobotomies and deep sleep therapy[554], have all been justified by grossly exaggerated claims of breakthroughs in brain science and technology. Although less dramatic than brain butchery, and repeated electroconvulsive therapy (ECT) while in extended drug induced comas, current 'drug first' psychiatric practices prematurely end or destroy many lives.

Too often, psychiatric drugs deliver short-term symptom relief at the expense of the long-term welfare of the patient. Too often, these drugs are prescribed for the benefit of everyone but the patient (e.g. the widespread use of antipsychotics to pacify annoying dementia patients in aged care facilities).

Psychiatry should protect vulnerable and distressed human beings and is meant to be based on robust science. It is the only profession that has the authority to involuntarily detain and drug people who have committed no crime. It needs to be held to a very high standard. Even higher than other medical disciplines. Instead, too often, psychiatry acts for the profit and convenience of the powerful at the expense of the disempowered.

There are many competent mental health practitioners who avoid the 'sugar-rush'-like benefits of the 'pills first ask questions later' approach; however, these responsible professionals have far too little influence on psychiatric practice. Sadly, the good that they do is often dwarfed by the harm caused by reckless prescribers.

Part of the problem is that critics of the dominance of drug treatments are playing on an uneven field. Take ADHD for example. Apart from a few determined and isolated sceptics, the high-profile experts in ADHD are almost exclusively fervent believers in the validity of the diagnosis and the safety and effectiveness of the drugs. These ADHD experts generally make a very good living specialising in diagnosing and treating ADHD or conducting drug company-sponsored research. Sceptics, however, cannot specialise or become recognised experts in conditions they do not believe in. It is impossible to make a comfortable living specialising in *not* diagnosing a condition.

This translates into research. I know from lived experience that it is next to impossible to attract research dollars for projects that don't reinforce the ADHD Industry's position. On the other hand, there are substantial incentives, both financial and professional, for 'true believers' who conduct industry friendly research ADHD. The pharmaceutical companies make sure their allies, both clinicians and 'patient support groups', are well resourced and rewarded. Critics, as I can personally attest, fight back as amateurs, with predictable results.

It is even worse for self-described 'psychiatric survivors' who have suffered ongoing harm from exposure to drugs, particularly antipsychotics. Often their criticisms of the impact of the drugs are dismissed as being attributable to their mental illness. When the opinions of 'psychiatric experts' compete with the opinions of diagnosed 'schizophrenics' (an almost impossible to lose label), the results are predictable.

Another significant driver of the drug dominant approach is that our current mental health services are located within general health services, be they GP surgeries or public hospitals. This reinforces the dominance of the medical model. The worst example is the fact that extremely unwell psychiatric patients in crisis are most often taken to busy, loud, brightly lit, crowded hospital emergency departments and are drugged by strangers. Could you design a less therapeutic environment for floridly psychotic, and often deeply traumatised, patients?

For their part, doctors, other mental health professionals and policy makers, who genuinely want to see better sustained outcomes from Australia's mental health system, need to restrict psychiatric practice to genuinely evidence-based parameters. This will require the Australian medical and psychiatric professions to acknowledge how little we actually know about the interplay between brain, body, biochemistry and behaviour. This in turn requires far greater respect for just how difficult the science and profession of psychiatry is.

Non-expert practitioners, especially GPs without extensive psychiatric and psychopharmacological training, should not be able to initiate psychotropic drug treatments. Most importantly, if a doctor is not capable of helping people withdraw from a mental health drug (usually by tapering), they should not be allowed to prescribe them. This would see fewer drugs being prescribed, and less profit made, particularly by Big Pharma. It would also mean less business for run-of-the-mill GPs.

The trend towards increasing reliance on drug treatments over psychotherapy has been further exacerbated by the growing dominance of corporatised multi-clinician practices in both the USA and Australia.[555] They have increased the emphasis on billable throughput and profit maximisation, in contrast to single clinician practices which enable personal patient relationships and profit satisficing (making a sufficient rather than maximised return). This has increased the pressure to diagnose early, with often the only approved treatments being pharmacological.[556]

The current dominance of the medical model is further reinforced by the way the efficiency of first-world health systems are measured.

The emphasis is on a cost-per-case basis over a fixed period of time. Cost-per-case cost means the number of cases of a particular type that are transacted per dollar within a fixed period of time (usually a week, month or year). Measured this way, the most efficient systems – which in turn become the most profitable – are those that conduct the highest number of transactions per dollar of expenditure within an accounting period. Accounting systems do not identify the long-term outcomes of treatments. For example, a psychiatric service that processes twice the number of patients per thousand dollars of public funding than another psychiatric service will be regarded as more efficient, regardless of the long-term outcomes for patients.

Adding to the superficial appeal of drugs over less interventionist treatments is the fact that the pathways of illness and the consequences of iatrogenic harm are often difficult to distinguish. This is particularly true for mental health patients, as many psychotropic drugs have the potential to either exacerbate pre-existing problems or create new problems.[557] This creates confusion in regard to cause and effect, where the iatrogenic effects are misinterpreted as the next step in the progression of mental illness. This can lead to increased dosage in a mistaken attempt to obtain the desired therapeutic effect, or the introduction of new pharmaceutical interventions, with potential additional side effects, to control the new problem.

The 'cause and effect' burden of proof in relation to iatrogenic harm prevents litigation being an effective deterrent for negligent iatrogenic damage. Although it may be relatively easy in population-based research to establish that a particular treatment carries a particular risk, establishing that it was the cause of an adverse outcome in an individual case is much more difficult. In addition, the unclear distinction between the pathway of disease and iatrogenic harm referred to above makes it very difficult for a plaintiff to establish that the treatment decision was unreasonable. For example, dexamphetamine and Ritalin both carry boxed warnings of their potential for addiction and abuse from prolonged use.[558] However, many ADHD proponents attribute drug abuse to being a consequence of the patient's ADHD rather than an iatrogenic consequence of prolonged use of these amphetamine-like substances.[559]

Medical regulation and review is largely regulated internally by the medical profession. The rationale for self-regulation is that only clinicians have the required expertise to judge the appropriateness of medical treatments. Although the argument has some validity, self-regulation carries the danger that there will be a closed culture of protecting the profession from external scrutiny and criticism.

Unlike the US, Australia does not allow direct advertising to consumers. To get around the ban on advertising specific drugs to consumers, Big Pharma sponsors disease awareness campaigns. Sometimes this happens through industry organisations like Medicines Australia, where individual pharmaceutical companies pool resources for their common interest. Sometimes they sponsor consumer organisations to help 'paint a picture of an under-diagnosed medical disorder best treated with drugs'.[560]

These consumer groups, however, are usually not puppets of the drug companies. Rather, drug companies partner with consumer groups with compatible positions on depression, anxiety, psychosis or ADHD. Only their motivations differ: the pharmaceutical companies seek profits and share price increases; the support groups are convinced they are helping children and families.

The restrictions on direct promotion to consumers do not apply to potential prescribers. The pharmaceutical industry aggressively markets its drugs to Australian doctors. By controlling the definitions of the disorders they diagnose through the DSM, and providing time-poor GPs (who do most of the prescribing) with a distorted picture of the risks and benefits of drug treatments, Big Pharma and Pseudo-Scientific Biological Psychiatry dominate psychiatric practise.

The development of the DSM and its dominant role in modern psychiatric practice also reflects broader changes in society. While most Australians are more prosperous than previous generations, the pace of life has accelerated, and the vast majority are now time poor. As a result, we increasingly want quick fixes. Drugs generally change things very quickly. It may not be a conscious decision, but we value short-term symptom management and often choose to assume that, if something helps now, it will also do us good in the long-term. For example, giving disruptive children a diagnostic label (e.g. ADHD) and a pill, and then seeing them immediately quieter and more compliant, seems like a win for all. Biological Psychiatry's seductive promise of a 'pill for every ill' is very hard to compete with.

Judged using short-term efficiency criteria, that is, the speed and dollar cost of processing large numbers of patients, the DSM framework performs well. It enables the increasingly dominant high patient throughput pattern of applying diagnostic labels and prescribing matched pharmaceutical interventions. Iatrogenic harm is often very hard to tie directly to a specific treatment.

There are also incentives for government to not acknowledge the shortcomings of the services they provide. The failure of clinical judgements by clinicians working in government run mental health systems is a consequence of decisions of individual clinicians. However, there are significant political risks for governments when these clinical failures are revealed. As a consequence, there may be a political penalty for governments seeking to expose failure within their own system. This can lead to a defensive culture of limiting exposure to information about iatrogenic events.

This tendency can be further enhanced by the political and industrial power of professional associations/unions like the Australian Medical Association and, to a lesser extent, the Australian Nursing Federation. In defence of their membership, they can blame inadequate government resourcing for the failings of individual clinicians and practitioners working within public systems.

The aim of modern health systems should be to maximise patient and societal wellbeing. This is not achieved by minimising iatrogenic harm but rather by undertaking all treatments with a positive benefit-risk profile. Inevitably this will involve some iatrogenic harm, and even iatrogenic deaths, in situations where an objective prospective analysis indicated the risk was 'worth taking'.

Unlike the airline industry, the mental health system does not aim to prevent all adverse events. However, there are lessons that can be learned from the forensic approach taken to investigating air crashes. Air crashes are unambiguously negative public events. Iatrogenic harm is often difficult to identify and therefore has the potential to be under-estimated and even wilfully ignored. The detail of iatrogenic events needs to be made public so that proper benefit/risk assessments can be made.

Mandatory, rather than voluntary, reporting of all suspected adverse events, to provide a more comprehensive database, would help to identify treatments requiring further investigation. This would need to be supplemented with independent, comprehensive, random sampling of short- and long-term treatment outcomes to determine the true extent of benefits and iatrogenic harm. In summary, developing effective accounting practices that recognise true benefits and iatrogenic harms is central to maximising individual and societal welfare.

Toby Hall, the Chief Executive Officer of the not-for-profit community support organisation Mission Australia, and a member of the Mental Health Expert Working Group established to advise the Australian Government on mental health, believes that the further medicalisation of mental distress must be resisted:

> Put simply our mental health system must move from delivering
> pills to delivering practical support and care built around
> fundamental needs such as employment and housing…while
> well-meaning, [the medical experts behind EPPIC and headspace
> and other initiatives] are trained to fix health issues not provide
> guidance on housing, skills training, accessing employment
> or enrolling in education. The solution is to put care ahead of
> medical treatment.[561]

Clearly our drug dominant approach isn't working. But, too often,
this fact seems lost on the decision makers who control the purse strings
and determine where our mental health dollars are spent. The best they
offer is more of what has already failed, and arguably worse still, driven
us backwards. It is well past the time for real evidence – not the wishful
thinking of mental health gurus/entrepreneurs – to guide mental health
policy and practice.

Professor Patrick McGorry and Professor Ian Hickie have been
Australia's two most influential mental health policy entrepreneurs in
the 21st century and have done a lot to make mental health a prominent
issue on the national political agenda.[562] Earlier in their careers, they
received significant financial support from Big Pharma. However, they
have outgrown the need for pharmaceutical industry funding, and
they now get most of the tens of millions they and their programs need
from government. Nonetheless, the seed funding invested early by Big
Pharma has proved a very astute investment.

Both McGorry and Hickie frequently argue the need for a radical
rethink of mental health policy and practice. They are correct, radical
change is needed. But the reforms they have driven appear to be
making a bad situation worse. The fundamental problem is that they
massively overstate what a mental health system can achieve. They argue

for a system that targets everyone from the severely psychotic to the moderately depressed, and even those perceived to be at mildly elevated risk of future mental illness. They have ignored contradictory evidence, and they vigorously point the finger of blame elsewhere, while escaping accountability for the poor outcomes that have occurred as their influence has risen.

Time for our elected leaders to stop following

Over the last decade and a half, successive Australian Commonwealth Governments, and some state governments, have made mental health reform a priority and have committed considerable resources. Yet, despite governments spending billions of dollars on new programs, and massive efforts to raise awareness, reduce stigma and intervene early, just about every measure of mental wellbeing has either not improved or has gone from bad to worse. Put simply, we are spending more to achieve less. Rates of diagnosis and treatment have jumped, but outcomes are going backwards. The most affected are children, teenagers and young adults. They are more likely than ever to be mentally ill and to suicide and self-harm.

This decline has happened as high profile, taxpayer funded, mental health organisations, particularly Beyond Blue, headspace, Orygen and SANE have emerged. Over the last twenty years, these organisations – some driven by home-grown, media savvy psychiatric thought leaders – have enjoyed the bipartisan support from our elected leaders and have grown enormously.

If we are to achieve better mental health outcomes, our elected leaders need to stop following failed experts. We need our nation's leaders to take the time to consider the independent, robust evidence and not be swayed by those with programs to promote, and empires to build. Prime Minister Morrison is still relatively new. Unlike Rudd,

Gillard, Abbott and Turnbull, he is secure from challenge from his own side. As detailed in chapter 2, Prime Minister Morrison, more than those who have gone before him, has made reducing youth suicide one of the key criteria against which he will be judged. By backing the architects of past failure, he made a very poor start. However, he has the time and the authority to change direction. If he continues to back failure, he must be held accountable.

Of course, the Commonwealth Government shares responsibility with eight individual state and territory governments. The Commonwealth Government has prime responsibility for:

- Ensuring that medications and medical products are safe and effective – through the Therapeutic Goods Administration.
- Subsidising medications via the Pharmaceutical Benefits Scheme (PBS).
- Primary and specialist diagnostic and treatment services (i.e. visits to GPs, psychiatrists, paediatricians, psychologists etc.).
- Working with the relevant professions and consumers to develop evidence-based diagnosis and treatment guidelines.
- Regulation of aged care services.

State and territory governments:

- Run public hospitals and public child, adolescent and adult mental health clinics and crisis care facilities.
- Run schools and police services and provide public housing.
- Run child welfare and protection services.

The interface between the Commonwealth and state governments in health and mental health has long been problematic. There is a long history of cost shifting and blame shifting between jurisdictions. This has usually involved one level of government creating barriers to entry, or incentives to exit, that encourage patients to move from services funded by them to services provided by the other level of government. The most common points of potential cost shifting are between the state government-funded hospitals, especially emergency departments, and Commonwealth Government-subsidised GPs and aged care facilities.

In recent years, the Commonwealth Government has bucked this trend and directly funded headspace and the McGorry inspired *Early Psychosis Services* targeted at 12- to 25-year-olds. This demographic has in the past been serviced by state-run child and adolescent services (for those aged under 18), or adult mental health services. The Commonwealth Government's direct intervention has created obvious duplication and coordination issues where siloed services may not interact effectively.

Victorian Royal Commission

The most striking example of the extraordinary influence McGorry has with both sides of politics was the decision by the Andrews Labor Victorian State Government to establish a Royal Commission into Mental Health and appoint McGorry as the Chair of the eight-member Expert Advisory Committee. The Royal Commission's Terms of Reference include investigating 'how to most effectively prevent mental illness and suicide'.[563] McGorry, through his leading roles at Orygen, headspace and EPYS, is a significant player in the Victorian mental health system as well as the Commonwealth mental health system. The Royal Commission should have been free to investigate, without fear or favour, the activities of McGorry and the programs and treatments he promotes.

If the Victorian Government was serious about tackling suicide, the Royal Commission should have investigated the impact of the advice offered by McGorry, Orygen, headspace, Hickie etc. It is absurd that a major player like McGorry advises the Royal Commission. It robs the Commission of credibility on these issues. The Andrews Government has also committed to implement every recommendation of the Royal Commission, before they have even been made. Why would any government commit to doing that, unless it knew in advance what the recommendations are likely to be?

With McGorry advising the Royal Commission, we can expect the Commission will recommend more money for his pet projects like EPYS. The truth is we would not fund EPYS if we were not defining mildly troubled young people as being pre-psychotic. Similarly, we wouldn't have such a problematic amphetamine culture if we didn't give so many inattentive and impulsive children (and an increasing number of adults) a daily amphetamine habit to manage their behaviour. Most troubling is the compelling evidence that indicates we might not need as many coffins for our young if we took the FDA suicide warnings and the Australian statistical data about antidepressant use and youth suicide seriously.

The limitations of mental health systems

Perhaps the bravest thing that politicians need to do is to own up to the limitations of government and the limitations of mental health interventions. They need to challenge the expectation that governments can alleviate, and even prevent, persistent unhappiness, anxiety and distress. Instead they are enabling unrealistic expectations of the capacity of government by engaging in bidding wars for the support of mental health gurus with insatiable appetites for taxpayer's dollars. Even governments of the Centre Right are buying into the nonsense that it is their job to spend taxpayer's money achieving the unachievable.

Of course there is a role for government, but good governments know their limits. Good governments foster tolerance and inclusion and help the disadvantaged live dignified lives, with the opportunity for improvement. Good governments also make sure that those with real debilitating mental illness get support that helps them recover, or at least live their best lives. Good governments are concerned about the long-term wellbeing of people, not quick (political or treatment) fixes.

Governments concerned about long-term patient wellbeing need to recognise there are three superficial reasons drugs appear more attractive than psychosocial treatments. First, psychological interventions are often more resource intensive in the short to medium term. Second, drugs usually alter behaviour much faster than non-drug treatments, and trials most often measure improvements in short-term symptom management (often for no longer than a few weeks). Third, the vast majority of psychiatric treatment research is funded by drug companies, with the emphasis on short-term effects rather than lasting benefits and harms. Consequently, pharmaceutical interventions are seriously over-rated and over-utilised.

To address this imbalance, Australian Governments, primarily the Commonwealth Government, but also state governments, should initiate multiple reforms.

Fifteen reforms needed in Australia to improve mental health outcomes

1. **Public disclosure of safety and efficacy data**. Massive reform of our system of regulating medical product safety and efficacy is required. The Australian Government, through the Pharmaceutical Benefits Scheme, has powerful levers to pull. It should make it a condition of licencing and subsidising pharmaceuticals and medical devices that there is full public disclosure of all safety and efficacy data held by product manufacturers (with protections for intellectual property and commercially sensitive costing information). There should be very heavy penalties, including immediate removal from market and massive fines (and possibly jail time for directors), for failing to disclose relevant information. Only product manufacturers who are not confident in the safety of their products would choose to take them off the market rather than expose the truth to public scrutiny.

2. **Prevent cherry picking of favourable results** by requiring pre-registration of all new research that may be later used to support the TGA licencing and PBS subsidisation of pharmaceutical products in Australia. Obviously this system would only work prospectively, and would not enable access to studies already concluded. To address this shortfall, details of all research conducted on a particular drug should be provided to the relevant regulator for consideration and made available for public scrutiny. This would help to address the problem of a narrow base of selective research used to licence and subsidise drugs. Regulators would have access to all related research. This would prevent a repeat of the situation which happened with Strattera, where research conducted by the drug manufacturer Eli Lilly was not made publicly available or provided to the relevant regulator because, without external scrutiny, the manufacturer determined it was not relevant.

3. **FOI Reform**. For this to happen, it would be necessary to reform Commonwealth Freedom of Information legislation to end the entitlement of corporations to rely on privacy provisions originally intended to protect the health records of individuals. The Commonwealth Government should also make adverse drug event reporting to the TGA for a specified range of serious reactions (suicidal ideation, strokes, psychosis etc.) mandatory, and regularly publish full de-identified details on the TGA website.

4. **Full public disclosure of pharmaceutical industry funding** sources for clinicians, researchers, patient groups, advisory board members and members of committees involved in regulatory and policy development processes is also required. The

Commonwealth Government should look at the US *Physician Payments Sunshine Act, passed in 2010 and co-sponsored by Republican Senator Chuck Grassley and Democrat Senator* Richard Blumenthal. The goal of the *Physician Payments Sunshine Act* was to increase the transparency of financial relationships between doctors and other health care providers and drug companies. Potential conflicts of interest should be made public. It was not perfect legislation, but at least it was a start.

5. **Consumer medicine information leaflets**. In addition, the Commonwealth Government should also strengthen Consumer Medicine Information (CMI) requirements, so that:

    *   Every warning currently included in information to prescribers is also on the CMI. (Currently warnings are often only highlighted on information made available to prescribers and are not seen by consumers.)

    *   It should also be mandatory to include a CMI inside medication packaging.

    *   A brief summary of the most serious safety warnings is written on the outside packaging of drugs, so consumers are aware of very significant risks.

6. **Off label prescribing** is another massive issue the Commonwealth Government needs to tackle. It should commission or conduct research into the incidence and impact of off label prescribing. The research should concentrate on the health impacts of off label prescribing and the extent of PBS subsidisation for the off label use of medications. Based on the outcome of this research, the Commonwealth Government may consider whether, over time, it would be worth encouraging off label prescribing to

become 'on label'. This could be achieved by gradually enforcing PBS subsidisation of medications to those prescribed within the approved guidelines. This might encourage pharmaceutical companies to apply to the TGA to expand the range of authorised uses of their products, and would help ensure that prescribing practices are supported by robust evidence.

7. **Without further delay, implement real-time electronic monitoring of pharmaceutical dispensing**. As discussed in Chapter 8, the Commonwealth and State Governments need to roll-out, without further delay (originally planned for 2012), the Electronic Recording and Reporting of Controlled Drugs (ERRCD) initiative. ERRCD would provide a mandatory, real-time, electronic tool for all pharmacies dispensing Controlled Drugs. Pharmacists would have real-time information from a database about previous dispensing episodes, enabling them to detect doctor shoppers.[564]

8. **Coordination of Commonwealth and State Government Spending**. In total, Australia will spend roughly $10 billion on mental health services in 2020. The State governments and the Commonwealth Government will contribute roughly equal proportions, with private health insurance providing the remaining 5%.[565] This is a lot of money, but we can have little confidence we are getting value for money. The Commonwealth and the States need to sort out the mishmash in service delivery. The practice of successive Federal Governments going it alone by directly funding services like headspace and *EPYS*, without robust supporting evidence, or regard for how these services integrate with state government services, should end. Too often, funding for these services has been based on short-term political

considerations and personal relationships with charismatic mental health gurus. This is just not how public policy should be done.

9. **Replace DSM with ICD.** One of the simpler reforms governments could initiate is to restrict financial support (including Medicare co-payments and PBS drug subsidisation) for the treatment of mental health disorders to those diagnosed using the World Health Organization's (WHO) ICD criteria. This would help end the dominance of the American Psychiatric Association's DSM criteria. Australia is a member of the WHO but has no capacity to influence the American Psychiatric Association. Alternatively, given that there are also concerns about the capture of WHO processes, Australia could develop its own diagnostic framework.

10. **Protect the human rights of involuntary patients**. State governments need to increase the protections or involuntary patients. Involuntary patients have, in the majority of cases, not committed any crime. Too many are detained and drugged against their will on a flimsy basis. Yes, it is legitimate to protect the public from dangerously psychotic individuals and self-harming patients; however, too often, patients are detained and drugged on vague grounds (e.g. to protect their reputation).

11. **Make adverse drug event reporting for a specified range of serious reactions (suicidal ideation, strokes, psychosis etc.) mandatory,** and regularly publish full details on the TGA website. Voluntary reporting means that only a tiny fraction of adverse events ever get reported. Arguably, reckless prescribers may be less likely to report serious adverse events than cautious prescribers because they may be concerned about acknowledging the consequences of their prescribing practices. The public has a right to know, and policy makers need to know about

the frequency of adverse events, so they can make informed decisions about the risk-benefit profile of medications.

12. **Prohibit pharmaceutical company donations to political parties and candidates and compensate if necessary through increased public funding of political parties.** Governments are responsible for multi-million-dollar decisions about which drugs get approved and subsidised, and must make these decisions without fear or favour. There is currently retrospective disclosure of political donations, and there is no evidence of direct corruption. However, there has been very little scrutiny of pharmaceutical company operations by parliamentarians. Although a similar case could be made for a range of industries, the pharmaceutical industry is unique, in that it produces mind and body altering chemicals that are ingested by children – a particularly vulnerable consumer group. Many of these chemical interventions are lifesaving; most are warranted but, as with ADHD, some are highly questionable. Government must be free from improper influence by the pharmaceutical industry.

13. **Address the inequity of resourcing of competing perspectives on controversial mental health and health policy issues by direct government funding of independent non-government pharmaceutical and medical/psychiatric watchdogs.** The pharmaceutical industry has demonstrated that it has sufficient resources to effectively organise, lobby and market to enhance its own economic interests. However, there is no significant counterbalancing economic interest that supports those concerned about the inappropriate and unsafe use of pharmacological interventions. Industry domination of notional consumer support groups further exacerbates the problem of regulatory capture by

creating the false impression of independent consumer-driven advocacy. Governments could address this imbalance by funding independent non-government watchdogs specifically tasked with critiquing research and clinical practice in the medical/psychiatric and pharmaceutical fields.

14. **Ensure diverse views are robustly represented in health and mental health policy and regulatory process.** In many cases, these types of processes (e.g. treatment guidelines development and drug prescribing oversight processes) are dominated by like-minded, industry friendly 'experts' who develop consensus (often unanimous outcomes). These processes should be open and contested, with a range of views competing to influence outcomes. Very often 'experts' in a single condition or disorder have significant financial or even intellectual and ideological conflicts of interest. [566] If medical knowledge is required to evaluate evidence of the safety and efficacy of treatments etc., this can generally be done by medical practitioners/researchers who don't specialise in the condition or disorder.

15. **Stop schools demanding that students be medicated as a condition of attendance.** There are too many disturbing reports of schools suggesting that a child has a psychiatric disorder, particularly ADHD, or, worse still, demanding that a child be 'medicated' (i.e. drugged with amphetamine) as a condition of attending school. This is a child rights abuse. It is particularly disturbing because, as detailed in Chapter 5, many children are drugged because schools and teachers mistake age-related immaturity, among the youngest in class, for a psychiatric disorder.

Although Australian politicians have shown little interest in tackling the influence of Big Pharma, there has been greater recognition of the problem in some other countries. In 2004–5, in response to concerns about the impact of inappropriate pharmaceutical industry influence on medical and psychiatric practice, the United Kingdom House of Commons established a Committee to conduct an inquiry titled *The Influence of the Pharmaceutical Industry Fourth Report of Session 2004–05.*[567]

Conclusions of the House of Commons Committee Inquiry into The Influence of the Pharmaceutical Industry Fourth Report of Session 2004–05

- Our over-riding concerns are about the volume, extent and intensity of the industry's influence, not only on clinical medicine and research but also on patients, regulators, the media, civil servants and politicians...

- The regulatory system, the medical profession and Government have all failed to ensure that industry's activities are more clearly allied to the interests of patients and the National Health Service.

- The influence of the pharmaceutical industry is such that it dominates clinical practice, to an extent that deprives it of independent and constructively critical feedback; this is a discipline it needs and which can help it to improve.

- The traditional secrecy in the drug regulatory process has insulated regulators from the feedback that would otherwise check, test and stimulate their policies and performance.

- The closeness that has developed between regulators and companies has deprived the industry of rigorous quality control and audit.

- Other bodies are in a position to provide feedback and

quality control. They include academic, research, clinical and professional institutions, as well as the media and patient groups. However, representatives of these interests have had only limited success in containing excessive industry influence. This can be partly attributed to lack of transparency, limited resources, significant dependency on industry funding, and some conflicts of interest.

The report detailed 'problems with SSRIs antidepressants, notably Seroxat, and the COX-2 inhibitors, Vioxx and Celebrex'. It found unethical behaviour by drug manufacturers in failing to disclose adverse information when applying to licence new drugs. However, it also found that 'prescribers must take their share of the blame for the problems that have resulted' as some 'medicines have been indiscriminately prescribed on a grand scale'. It attributed this reckless prescribing to 'intensive promotional activity' and 'data secrecy and uncritical acceptance of drug company views'.[568]

The Committee concluded that the consequences of the above-mentioned failings were the 'unsafe use of drugs' and 'increasing medicalisation of society'. They also found that the 'drift towards medicalisation is a global phenomenon', and concluded that, despite the problems identified above, the 'UK may have a better record than many others [countries]'. The Committee made a number of specific recommendations to tackle what it termed a 'pill for every ill' culture 'compounded by an excessive reliance on results from premarketing clinical trials, together with a failing system of pharmacovigilance'.[569] Given the cultural and institutional similarities between Australia and the United Kingdom, the House of Commons Committee's conclusions and recommendations may have relevance in Australia. Several of my fifteen recommendations are similar to those made by that Committee.

In 2018, in recognition of the need to move away from the 'pill for every ill' approach, the UK Government appointed its first Minister for Loneliness.[570] Most people in the UK aged over 75 live alone, and it was estimated in 2018 that about 200,000 older people in the UK had not had a conversation with a friend or relative in more than a month.[571] However, this epidemic of loneliness is not limited to the elderly, as the highest rate of self-reported loneliness in the UK is among those aged 16 to 24 years.[572] Whether a government can help prevent its citizens being lonely and sad is a valid question, and there are already plans to turn loneliness into a discrete psychiatric disorder treated with drugs[573], but at least the initiative of appointing a Minister for Loneliness reflects an understanding of one of the social drivers of well-being.

Many of the fifteen reforms suggested above would require courageous political leadership, something we have not seen in Australian federal politics for a very long time. A significant barrier to these necessary reforms will be the influence of the pharmaceutical industry and their peak body, Medicines Australia. Big Pharma's enormous economic resources and political skills have enabled them to dominate, virtually uncontested, the processes of licencing and subsidising their products in Australia. Without political leadership on these issues, Australians will continue to be denied fully informed consent and be exposed to unnecessary risks.

For their part, doctors, other mental health professionals and policy makers who genuinely want to see better sustained outcomes Australia's mental health system, need to restrict psychiatric practice to robust evidence-based parameters. This will require the Australian medical and psychiatric professions to acknowledge how little they actually know about the interplay between brain, body, biochemistry and behaviour. This in turn requires far greater respect for just how difficult it is to be a competent, empathetic psychiatrist, who knows both their patients the relevant science.

Psychiatry is an exceptionally difficult and complex profession that must be done by highly skilled specialists. Non-expert practitioners, especially GPs without extensive psychiatric and psychopharmacological training, should not be able to initiate psychotropic drug treatments. Most importantly, if a doctor is not capable of helping people withdraw from a mental health drug (usually by tapering), they should not be allowed to prescribe them.

Government and the psychiatric and medical professions and even the media need to lift their game. But ultimately the Madmen marketing us our epidemic of mental illness couldn't sell their products if consumers were not buying.

Clinicians and patients in developed nations like Australia typically have a provider-customer relationship. There is often an expectation by consumers that a successful consultation results in a diagnosis and prescription. The patient may believe that the transaction is incomplete or does not represent value for both time and money if a definite product does not result. In the eyes of many patients, a clinician who recommends watchful waiting, and does not provide a diagnosis and treatment, is not doing their job properly.

If we want improved mental wellbeing, the most obvious change that needs to happen is that patients need to stop believing in 'quick fixes'. Pills may work in the short term, and for a minority of severely ill patients they may be required for extended periods, but very often they do much more harm than good in the long run.

Patients and parents need to stop expecting that they can take a pill to resolve their or their child's problems. They need to remember that if something sounds too good to be true...

Endnotes

1   Tony Bartone, President Australian Medical Association, Ian Hickie Brain and Mind Centre, Patrick McGorry Orygen, Centre for Youth Mental Health. Joint Statement: Covid-19 impact likely to lead to increased rates of suicide and mental illness, 7 May 2020, https://ama.com.au/media/joint-statement-covid-19-impact-likely-lead-increased-rates-suicide-and-mental-illness (accessed 14 August 2020).

2   Brad Ryan, Celina Edmonds and Sophie Scott, Coronavirus pandemic plan for mental health too small, suicides likely to increase, expert says. ABC News, 15 May 2020, https://www.abc.net.au/news/2020-05-15/coronavirus-pandemic-mental-health-package-reaction/12253820 (accessed 6 June 2020).

3   Whitely M (2011) Hansard Western Australian Parliament [25 May 2011 pp. 3984d-3994a. Available at: http://www.parliament.wa.gov.au/Hansard/hansard.nsf/0/75032653ddacbe7f482578b100299ab4/$FILE/A38+S1+20110525+p3984d-3994a.pdf (accessed 11 February 2019).

4   In the 2018/9 financial year, 4.3 million Australians were prescribed at least one mental health medication. Australian Institute of Health and Welfare. Mental Health Services in Australia, 30 Jan 2020, https://www.aihw.gov.au/reports/mental-health-services/mental-health-services-in-australia/report-contents/mental-health-related-prescriptions (accessed 1 June 2020).

5   Whitely M.1 in 8 (over 3 million) Australians are on antidepressants — Why is the Lucky Country so miserable? PsychWatch Australia Blog. April 2019 available at https://www.psychwatchaustralia.com/post/1-in-8-over-3-million-australians-are-on-antidepressants-why-is-the-lucky-country-so-miserable (accessed 1 June 2020).

6   Health at a Glance 2017: OECD Indicators Antidepressant drugs consumption, 2000 and 2015 (or nearest year) OECD Publishing 2017. Available at https://read.oecd-ilibrary.org/social-issues-migration-health/health-at-a-glance-2017/antidepressant-drugs-consumption-2000-and-2015-or-nearest-year_health_glance-2017-graph181-en#page1 (accessed 1 June 2020).

7   Depression and Other Common Mental Disorders: Global Health Estimates. Geneva: World Health Organization; 2017. Licence: CC BY-NC-SA 3.0 IGO Available at https://apps.who.int/iris/bitstream/handle/10665/254610/WHO-MSD-MER-2017.2-eng.pdf;jsessionid=4C3AC0DC58EEAF097117E33D3C9F4513?sequence=1 (accessed 16 April 2019).

8   Frances A. World's Best and Worst Places to Be Mentally Ill Neglecting and excluding the mentally ill makes their symptoms much worse. 28 December 2015. https://www.psychologytoday.com/us/blog/saving-normal/201512/worlds-best-and-worst-places-be-mentally-ill (accessed 29 June 2020).

9   Council of Australian Government Health Council 2017, The Fifth National Mental Health and Suicide Prevention. Available at http://www.coaghealthcouncil.gov.au/Portals/0/Fifth%20National%20Mental%20Health%20and%20Suicide%20Prevention%20Plan.pdf (accessed 17 November 2019).

10   Lauren Cook, Mental health in Australia: a quick guide, Parliament of Australia, Social Policy Section, 14 February 2019. Available at https://www.aph.gov.au/About_Parliament/Parliamentary_Departments/Parliamentary_Library/pubs/rp/rp1819/Quick_Guides/MentalHealth (accessed 3 January 2020).

11   https://www.aph.gov.au/About_Parliament/Parliamentary_Departments/Parliamentary_Library/pubs/rp/rp1819/Quick_Guides/MentalHealth

12   Tom Stayner, 'This has to change': Mental ill-health costs Australia $500 million every day. SBS News 31 October 2019. Available at https://www.sbs.com.au/news/this-has-to-change-mental-ill-health-costs-australia-500-million-every-day

13   Robert Whittaker, *Anatomy of an Epidemic: Magic Bullets, Psychiatric Drugs, and the Astonishing Rise of Mental Illness in America*. Crown Publishing Group (2010).

14   Whitely MP. Attention Deficit Hyperactivity Disorder Policy, Practice and Regulatory Capture in Australia 1992–2012 [PhD]. Perth, WA: Curtin University; 2014. https://espace.curtin.edu.au/bitstream/handle/20.500.11937/1776/225953_Whitely%202014.pdf?sequence=2&isAllowed=y (accessed 15 June 2020).

15   Australian Institute of Health and Welfare 2016. Mental health services — in brief 2016. Cat. no. HSE 180 Canberra: AIHW. pp. 24-25 Available at https://www.aihw.gov.au/getmedia/681f0689-8360-4116-b1cc-9d2276b65703/20299.pdf.aspx?inline=true (accessed 13 August 2018).

16   Australian Institute of Health and Welfare. Mental Health Services in Australia (2020). Available at https://www.aihw.gov.au/getmedia/584d7a31-7c4a-46cb-97db-a46874265354/Mental-health-related-prescriptions-2018-19.pdf.aspx (accessed 13 August 2018).

17   The global pharmaceutical market has experienced significant growth in recent years. As of 2018 the total global pharmaceutical market is valued at about 1.2 trillion U.S. dollars. This is a significant increase from 2001 when the market was valued at just 390 billion U.S. dollars. Available at https://www.statista.com/statistics/263102/pharmaceutical-market-worldwide-revenue-since-2001/

18   Tiash Saha, The biggest ever pharmaceutical lawsuits, 25 June 2019, Pharmaceutical Technology. Available at https://www.pharmaceutical-technology.com/features/biggest-pharmaceutical-lawsuits/ (accessed 13 August 2018).

19   Despite the recent slippage, Australians are ranked near the top of world happiness rankings (11th of 185 countries in 2019 down from 10th in 2018) Helliwell, J., Layard, R., & Sachs, J. (2019). World Happiness Report 2019, New York: Sustainable Development Solutions Network. Available at https://s3.amazonaws.com/happiness-report/2019/WHR19.pdf (accessed 2 June 2020).

20   Margot O'Neill, Premature deaths linked to drugs in nursing homes. ABC Lateline 16 August 2012. Available at https://www.abc.net.au/news/2012-08-17/dementia-patients-dying-as-anti-psychotic-drugs-over-prescribed/4204536 (accessed 1 June 2020).

21   Sarah Ison. Mum's prescription drug warning to parents, antidepressants led to 'obsession with death' The West Australian, 27 June 2019. Available at https://thewest.com.au/news/medicine/mums-prescription-drug-warning-to-parents-antidepressants-led-to-obsession-with-death-ng-b881242232z (accessed 1 June 2020).

22   Whitely M. More young Australians suicide/self-harm and use antidepressants while experts dismiss FDA warning. PsychWatch Australia (1 June 2019). Available at: https://www.psychwatchaustralia.com/post/more-young-australians-suicide-self-harm-and-use-antidepressants-while-experts-dismiss-fda-warning (accessed 20 November 2019).

23   Mark Abadi, Katie Warren. The 10 most liveable cities in the world in 2019. Business Insider Australia, 19 August 2018. Available at. https://www.businessinsider.com.au/most-livable-cities-in-the-world-2018-8?r=US&IR=T (accessed 2 June 2020).

24   Australian Government, Australian trade and Investment commission. Investor Update – Australia holds world record for longest period of growth among developed economies 28 November 2018 https://www.austrade.gov.au/international/invest/investor-updates/2018/australia-holds-world-record-for-longest-period-of-growth-among-developed-economies (accessed 29 June 2020).

25   Depression and Other Common Mental Disorders: Global Health Estimates. Geneva: World Health Organization; 2017. Licence: CC BY-NC-SA 3.0 IGO Available at https://apps.who.int/iris/bitstream/handle/10665/254610/WHO-MSD-MER-2017.2-eng.pdf;jsessionid=4C3AC0DC58EEAF097117E33D3C9F4513?sequence=1 (accessed 16 April 2019).

26   Miller S.G. 1 in 6 Americans Takes a Psychiatric Drug. Scientific American. 13 December 2016 https://www.scientificamerican.com/article/1-in-6-americans-takes-a-psychiatric-drug/ (accessed 1 June 2020).

27   Associated Press, Global study finds mental illness widespread, NBC News. http://www.nbcnews.com/id/5111202/ns/health-mental_health/t/global-study-finds-mental-illness-widespread/#.XVjE8OgzY2w (accessed 2 June 2020).

28   Centres for Disease Control, Data and Statistics About ADHD. https://www.cdc.gov/ncbddd/adhd/data.html (accessed 2 June 2020).

29   Sultan, R. S., Correll, C. U., Schoenbaum, M., King, M., Walkup, J. T., & Olfson, M. (2018). National Patterns of Commonly Prescribed Psychotropic Medications to Young People. Journal of child and adolescent psychopharmacology, 28(3), 158–165. https://www.ncbi.nlm.nih.gov/pmc/articles/PMC5905871/ (accessed 2 June 2020).

30   Lukton E. Which countries have the best literacy and numeracy rates? World Economic Forum, 3 February 2016. Available at https://www.weforum.org/agenda/2016/02/which-countries-have-the-best-literacy-and-numeracy-rates/ (accessed 2 June 2020).

31   Fiallo J. U.S. falls in world happiness report, Finland named happiest country - What are the happiest countries on earth, and why isn't the U.S. one of them? Tampa Bay Times .21 March 2019. https://www.tampabay.com/data/2019/03/20/us-falls-in-world-happiness-report-finland-named-happiest-country/ (accessed 2 June 2020).

32   Khazan O. Americans Are Dying Even Younger Drug overdoses and suicides are causing American life expectancy to drop. *The Atlantic*, 29 November 2018. https://www.theatlantic.com/health/archive/2018/11/us-life-expectancy-keeps-falling/576664/ (accessed 2 June 2020).

33   Whitely M.1 in 8 (over 3 million) Australians are on antidepressants — Why is the Lucky Country so miserable? PsychWatch Australia Blog. April 2019. https://www.psychwatchaustralia.com/post/1-in-8-over-3-million-australians-are-on-antidepressants-why-is-the-lucky-country-so-miserable (accessed 1 June 2020).

34   Whitely M, Raven M, Jureidini J. Antidepressant prescribing and suicide/self-harm by young Australians: Regulatory warnings, contradictory advice, and long-term trends. *Frontiers in Psychiatry* June 2020 https://www.frontiersin.org/articles/10.3389/fpsyt.2020.00478/full (accessed 1 June 2020).

35   Whitely M. 1 in 8 (over 3 million) Australians are on antidepressants — Why is the Lucky Country so miserable? PsychWatch Australia Blog. April 2019. https://www.psychwatchaustralia.com/post/1-in-8-over-3-million-australians-are-on-antidepressants-why-is-the-lucky-country-so-miserable (accessed 1 June 2020).

36   Drescher J, Out of DSM: Depathologizing Homosexuality, Behavorial Science (Basel). 2015 Dec; 5(4): 565–575. Available at https://www.ncbi.nlm.nih.gov/pmc/articles/PMC4695779/ (accessed 2 June 2020).

37   Allen Frances comments in 'Psychiatrists Propose Revisions to Diagnosis Manual', PBS Newshour, 10 February 2010. https://www.pbs.org/newshour/show/psychiatrists-propose-revisions-to-diagnosis-manual (accessed 2 June 2020).

38   'Psychiatry is more like a two-party political system with the biological [biomedicalized] and environmental parties constantly vying for power. Biological psychiatry is now the party in power.' Breggin P. Talking back to Ritalin: What doctors aren't telling you about stimulants for children, Common Courage Press. 1998 p.286.

39   NPR, Decoding 'the Most Complex Object in the Universe' Heard on Talk of the Nation. June 14, 2013. https://www.npr.org/2013/06/14/191614360/decoding-the-most-complex-object-in-the-universe (accessed 2 June 2020).

40   Randerson J. How many neurons make a human brain? Billions fewer than we thought. *The Guardian*. 28 February 2012. https://www.theguardian.com/science/blog/2012/feb/28/how-many-neurons-human-brain (accessed 2 June 2020).

41   Barkley R. *Taking Charge of ADHD*, Revised Edition: The Complete, Authoritative Guide. Guilford Publications 2000 p.272.

42   Guze, S. B. Biological psychiatry: Is there any other kind? *Psychological Medicine, 1989* 19(2), pp. 315-323.

43   Whitley Rob, Is psychiatry a religion? *Journal of the Royal Society of Medicine*. 1 December 2008; 101(12)579. https://www.ncbi.nlm.nih.gov/pmc/articles/PMC2625374/ (accessed 29 June 2020).

44   How do medications treat mental illness? Medications work by rebalancing the chemicals in the brain. Different types of medication act on different chemical pathways. https://www.yourhealthinmind.org/treatments-medication/medication (accessed 6 January 2020).

45   Australian Government Department of Health and Ageing: multiple brochures available at https://www1.health.gov.au/internet/publications/publishing.nsf/Content/mental-pubs-w-whatmen-toc~mental-pubs-w-whatmen-about (accessed 6 January 2020).

46   This brochure is part of a series on mental illness funded by the Australian Government under the National Mental Health Strategy…Australian Government Department of Health and Ageing: GPO Box 9848 CANBERRA ACT 2601What is a depressive disorder? https://www1.health.gov.au/internet/main/publishing.nsf/Content/01583965211717A9CA257BF0001E8D74/$File/whatdep2.pdf (accessed 6 January 2020).

47   Royal College of Psychiatrists (UK) Position statement on antidepressants and depression May 2019. https://www.rcpsych.ac.uk/docs/default-source/improving-care/better-mh-policy/position-statements/ps04_19---antidepressants-and-depression.pdf?sfvrsn=ddea9473_5 (accessed 29 June 2020).

48   Ian Hamilton. Are antidepressants addictive? This is what patients are telling us. Independent. 3 October 2019. https://www.independent.co.uk/voices/antidepressants-drugs-pills-opioids-addiction-mental-health-a9131901.html (accessed 29 June 2020).

49   Coslett R.L. I know antidepressant withdrawal symptoms are real. Why didn't doctors? *The*

Guardian, 30 May 2019. https://www.theguardian.com/commentisfree/2019/may/30/antidepressant-withdrawal-symptoms-doctors-side-effects (accessed 6 January 2020).

50   National Institute of Drug Abuse Stimulant ADHD Medications: Methylphenidate and Amphetamines. https://www.drugabuse.gov/publications/drugfacts/prescription-stimulants (accessed 2 June 2020).

51   Wang G.J. Long-Term Stimulant Treatment Affects Brain Dopamine Transporter Level in Patients with Attention Deficit Hyperactive Disorder. Published online 15 May 2013. https://www.ncbi.nlm.nih.gov/pmc/articles/PMC3655054/ (accessed 29 June 2020).

52   Steve Baldwin & Rebecca Anderson. The cult of methylphenidate: Clinical update, Critical Public Health, 10:1, pp. 81-86, 2000. https://www.tandfonline.com/doi/abs/10.1080/713658225 (accessed 29 June 2020).

53   Breggin P. Talking back to Ritalin: What doctors aren't telling you about stimulants for children, Common Courage Press. 1998 p.216.

54   Quoted in Breggin P. Talking back to Ritalin: What doctors aren't telling you about stimulants for children, Common Courage Press. 1998. p. 215.

55   Glenmullen J. *Prozac Backlash: Overcoming the Dangers of Prozac, Zoloft, Paxil, and other Antidepressants with Safe, Effective Alternatives,* Simon & Schuster, New York, 2000, p. 196.

56   *Gøtzsche P.* What are your burning issues for 2018? Psychiatry is a disaster area in healthcare that we need to focus on. BMJ 2018. 4 January 2018. https://www.bmj.com/content/360/bmj.k9/rr-15 (accessed 29 June 2020).

57   Respondents Urge Caution When Using the DSM-IV, *Clinical Psychiatry News*, 28(1): 14, 2000.

58   Cafasso J. Chemical Imbalance in the Brain: What you should know. Healthline. 4 December 2019. https://www.healthline.com/health/chemical-imbalance-in-the-brain?fbclid=IwAR1WCHrqK WxLHPKiGzxTQWDsdlk-GF-qLvl97EtqDbkbb52N6BsORL4egUU (accessed 2 June 2020).

59   Grand View Research. Market Research Report — Attention Deficit Hyperactivity Disorder (ADHD) Market Analysis Report by Drug Type (Stimulant, Non-stimulant), By Demographic, By Distribution Channel (Hospital & Retail Pharmacy), And Segment Forecasts, 2019 – 2025. February 2019, https://www.grandviewresearch.com/industry-analysis/attention-deficit-hyperactivity-disorder-adhd-market (accessed 29 June 2020).

60   International Monetary Fund. World Economic Outlook Database bit.ly/3dPAFmx (accessed 29 June 2020).

61   A Comparison of DSM-IV and DSM-5 Panel Members' Financial Associations with Industry: A Pernicious Problem Persists. Lisa Cosgrove , Sheldon Krimsky Plos Medicine March 13, 2012 https://journals.plos.org/plosmedicine/article?id=10.1371/journal.pmed.1001190 (accessed 29 June 2020).

62   Gardiner Harris and Benedict Carey, 'Psychiatric Group Faces Scrutiny Over Drug Industry Ties,' *The New York Times*, 12 July 2008. Available at https://www.nytimes.com/2008/07/12/washington/12psych.html (accessed 2 December 2019).

63   Steven S. Sharfstein, 'Big Pharma and American Psychiatry', Psychiatric News, Vol. 40, No. 16, August 2008, p. 3. Available at https://psychnews.psychiatryonline.org/doi/10.1176/pn.40.16.00400003 (accessed 2 December 2019).

64   Interview with Professor Allen Frances by Judy Woodruff, Psychiatrists Propose Revisions to Diagnosis Manual, PBS News Hour. 10 February 2010 12:00 AM EDT Transcript available at https://www.pbs.org/newshour/show/psychiatrists-propose-revisions-to-diagnosis-manual (Accessed 29 August 2019).

65   https://www.huffpost.com/entry/dsm-5_b_2227626

66   This is an edited version of a Huff Post blog written by Professor Allen Frances MD who is a Professor Emeritus of Psychiatry and former Chair at Duke University. DSM-5 Is a Guide, Not a Bible: Simply Ignore Its 10 Worst Changes. 12/03/2012 06:45 pm ET **Updated** Feb 02, 2013 https://www.huffpost.com/entry/dsm-5_b_2227626 (accessed 29 June 2019).

67   The Royal Australian College of Psychiatrists. Diagnostic Manuals – Position Statement 77, October 2016 https://www.ranzcp.org/news-policy/policy-and-advocacy/position-statements/diagnostic-manuals (accessed 29 June 2019).

68   Mahli G.S. et al. Royal Australian and New Zealand College of Psychiatrists clinical practice guidelines for mood disorders. https://www.ranzcp.org/files/resources/college_statements/clinician/cpg/mood-disorders-cpg.aspx (accessed 2 June 2020).

69   Rosemary F. Roberts, Kerry C. Innes & Susan M. Walker (1998), 'Introducing ICD-10-AM in Australian hospitals', Medical Journal of Australia, Medical Journal Australia, 169;8, pp.32-35. Available at https://www.mja.com.au/journal/1998/169/8/introducing-icd-10-am-australian-hospitals (accessed 2 May 2013).

70   Merete Juul Sorenson, Ole Mors and Per Hove Thomsen, 'DSM-IV or ICD-10-DCR diagnoses in child and adolescent psychiatry: does it matter?, European Journal of Child and Adolescent Psychiatry, 14; 6 (Sept 2005): p. 339. https://pubmed.ncbi.nlm.nih.gov/16220218/ (accessed 4 June 2006).

71   Whitely M.1 in 8 (over 3 million) Australians are on antidepressants — Why is the Lucky Country so miserable? PsychWatch Australia Blog. April 2019 available at https://www.psychwatchaustralia.com/post/1-in-8-over-3-million-australians-are-on-antidepressants-why-is-the-lucky-country-so-miserable (accessed 1 June 2020).

72   Sane Australia. Antipsychotic medication. Webpage https://www.sane.org/information-stories/facts-and-guides/antipsychotic-medication (accessed 2 June 2020).

73   Table PBS.2: Number of patients dispensed one or more mental health-related prescriptions, by type of medication prescribed and prescribing medical practitioner, states and territories, 2017–18 https://www.aihw.gov.au/reports/mental-health-services/mental-health-services-in-australia/report-contents/mental-health-related-prescriptions/interactive-data (accessed 29 June 2020).

74   Joel Magarey, Spike in number of Australian children put on antipsychotic drugs. News.com.au, 18 December 2018. https://www.news.com.au/lifestyle/health/health-problems/spike-in-number-of-australian-children-put-on-antipsychotic-drugs/news-story/4a4e4f373d3a98bdd5e8cfc66669e028#bottom-share (accessed 4 June 2020).

75   Cipriani A, Zhou X, Del Giovane C, Hetrick SE, Qin B, Whittington C, et al. Comparative efficacy and tolerability of antidepressants for major depressive disorder in children and adolescents: a network meta-analysis. Lancet (2016) 388(1047):881–90. doi: 10.1016/S0140-6736(16)30385-3 https://www.thelancet.com/journals/lancet/article/PIIS0140-6736(16)30385-3/fulltext (accessed 4 June 2020).

76   Safer DJ, Zito JM. Short- and Long-Term Antidepressant Clinical Trials for Major Depressive Disorder in Youth: Findings and Concerns. Frontiers in Psychiatry (2019) 10:705. doi: 10.3389/fpsyt.2019.0070512. https://www.frontiersin.org/articles/10.3389/fpsyt.2019.00705/full (accessed 4 June 2020).

77   Adverse Drug Reactions Advisory Committee, Use of SSRI antidepressants in children and adolescents, October 2004. Therapeutic Goods Administration. 15 October 2004. https://www.tga.gov.au/use-ssri-antidepressants-children-and-adolescents-october-2004 (accessed 29 June 2020).

78   Australian Commission on Safety and Quality in Healthcare, Website of the First Australian Atlas of Healthcare Variation 2015 Section 4 Interventions for mental health and psychotropic medicines Subsection 4.2 Antidepressant medicines dispensing 17 years and under. http://acsqhc.maps.arcgis.com/apps/MapJournal/index.html?appid=398ebb592c0a40cf913814bd7b965546# (accessed 29 June 2020).

79   Editorial, Prescribing off-label drugs for children: when will it change? The Lancet, September 28. https://www.thelancet.com/journals/lancet/article/PIIS0140-6736(19)32212-3/fulltext?dgcid=raven_jbs_etoc_email https://doi.org/10.1016/S0140-6736(19)32212-3 (accessed 29 June 2020).

80   Food and Drug Administration. Revisions to Product Labeling: Suicidality and Antidepressant Drugs. Rockville, MD: Food and Drug Administration (2004/2007). Available at: http://www.fda.gov/downloads/drugs/drugsafety/informationbydrugclass/ucm173233.pdf (accessed 16 March 2019).

81   Food and Drug Administration. Antidepressant Use in Children, Adolescents, and Adults. 2 May 2007. https://wayback.archive-it.org/7993/20171101224428/https:/www.fda.gov/Drugs/DrugSafety/InformationbyDrugClass/UCM096273 (accessed 15 April 2020).

82   Stone M, Laughren T, Jones ML, Levenson M, Holland PC, Hughes A, et al. (2009) Risk of suicidality in clinical trials of antidepressants in adults: analysis of proprietary data submitted to US Food and Drug Administration, BMJ (2009) 339:b2880. doi: 10.1136/bmj.b2880. p.431 https://www.bmj.com/content/339/bmj.b2880 (accessed 15 April 2020).

83   Friedman RA, Leon AC. Expanding the black box – depression, antidepressants, and the risk of suicide. New England Journal of Medicine (2007) 356(23):2343-6. https://www.nejm.org/doi/full/10.1056/nejmp078015 (accessed 4 June 2020).

84   Adverse Drug Reactions Advisory Committee (Therapeutic Goods Administration). Suicidality with SSRIs: adults and children. Australian Adverse Drug Reactions Bulletin (August 2005) 24(5). Available at: https://www.tga.gov.au/publication-issue/australian-adverse-drug-reactions-bulletin-vol-24-no-4#a1(accessed 19 November 2019).
85   Australian Government. Therapeutic Goods Amendment (Repeal of Ministerial Responsibility for Approval of RU486) Bill 2005. Community Affairs Legislation Committee (accessed 3 February 2006).
86   Suicide Prevention Australia Website Homepage. Available at: https://www. suicidepreventionaust.org (accessed 14 September 2019).
87   Suicide Prevention Australia Position statement: Youth Suicide Prevention (2010). p.17 Available until 5 March 2019 at: https://www.suicidepreventionaust.org/sites/default/files/resources/2016/SPA-Youth-Suicide-Prevention-Position-Statement%5B1%5D.pdf (accessed 4 March 2019).
88   "To our knowledge, there have been no psychopharmacological studies that have specifically targeted suicidal adolescents.(p.399)" Gould, M., Greenberg, T., Velting, D. & Shaffer, D. (2003a) 'Youth Suicide Risk and Prevention Interventions: A Review of the Last 10 Years'. *Journal of the American Academy of Child Adolescent Psychiatry 42*, 4, p.388 Available at https://health. maryland.gov/suicideprevention/Documents/Youth%20suicide%20risk%20and%20preventive%20 interventions-review%20of%20past%2010%20years.pdf (accessed 13 February 2019).
89   Suicide Prevention Australia Position statement: Youth Suicide Prevention 2010. p.17 Available until 5 March 2019 at: https://www.suicidepreventionaust.org/sites/default/files/resources/2016/SPA-Youth-Suicide-Prevention-Position-Statement%5B1%5D.pdf (accessed 4 March 2020).
90   Hetrick SE, Merry S, McKenzie J, Sindahl P, Proctor M. Selective Serotonin Reuptake Inhibitors (SSRIs) for Depressive Disorders in Children and Adolescents. Cochrane Database of Systematic Reviews. The Cochrane Library, Issue 3. (2007) Available at: https://www.ncbi.nlm.nih.gov/ pubmed/17636776 (accessed 12 March 2019).
91   Suicide Prevention Australia Position statement: Youth Suicide Prevention (2010). p.17 Available until 5 March 2019 p. 17 at: https://www.suicidepreventionaust.org/sites/default/files/resources/2016/ SPA-Youth-Suicide-Prevention-Position-Statement%5B1%5D.pdf (accessed 4 March 2020).
92   Hetrick SE, Merry S, McKenzie J, Sindahl P, Proctor M. Selective Serotonin Reuptake Inhibitors (SSRIs) for Depressive Disorders in Children and Adolescents. Cochrane Database of Systematic Reviews. The Cochrane Library, Issue 3. (2007) p. 29 Available at: https://www.ncbi.nlm.nih.gov/ pubmed/17636776 (accessed 12 March 2019).
93   Hetrick SE, Merry S, McKenzie J, Sindahl P, Proctor M. Selective Serotonin Reuptake Inhibitors (SSRIs) for Depressive Disorders in Children and Adolescents. Cochrane Database of Systematic Reviews. The Cochrane Library, Issue 3. (2007) p. 2 Available at: https://www.ncbi.nlm.nih.gov/ pubmed/17636776 (accessed 12 March 2019).
94   Northern Territory Parliamentary Website. Available at: https://parliament.nt.gov.au/__data/ assets/pdf_file/0008/366425/Sub-No.-20,-Suicide-Prevention-Australia,-Part-4,-6-Oct-2011.pdf (Accessed 17 November 2019).
95   Australian Bureau of Statistics, 3303.0 Causes of Death, Australia, 2019, Table 11.1 Intentional self-harm, Number of deaths, 5 year age groups by sex, 2010-2019. 23 October 2020 p.16 https://www. abs.gov.au/statistics/health/causes-death/causes-death-australia/latest-release
96   Suicide Prevention Australia Annual Financial Report for the year ending 30 June 2013. https:// acncpubfilesprodstorage.blob.core.windows.net/public/cd090126-38af-e811-a963-000d3ad244fd-5c76ba1f-b5cf-4fd3-8beb-bce4a508cd39-Financial%20Report-4f2efc3b-3eb0-e811-a962-000d3ad24a0d-SPA_-_Final_2013_annual_report.pdf (Accessed 29 June 2019).
97   Suicide Prevention Australia 2018/19 Annual Financial Report. https://www. suicidepreventionaust.org/wp-content/uploads/2019/11/2018-2019_Suicide-Prevention-Australia-Annual-Report.pdf (Accessed 29 June 2019).
98   Hetrick S, Purcell R. Evidence Summary: Using SSRI Antidepressants to Treat Depression in Young People: What are the Issues and What is the Evidence? Melbourne: Orygen Youth Health Research Centre 2009. Available at: https://web.archive.org/web/20130428063353/http://www. headspace.org.au/core/Handlers/MediaHandler.ashx?mediaId=4896 (Accessed 18 March 2019).
99   Orygen. Revolution in Mind, Annual Report 2018-2019. Available at https://www.orygen. org.au/getmedia/d88e0fc0-f773-46dd-9f70-33c1cc546fe8/Orygen_Annual_Report_2018-2019.aspx (Accessed 14 April 2020).

100   Hetrick S, Purcell R. Evidence Summary: Using SSRI Antidepressants to Treat Depression in Young People: What are the Issues and What is the Evidence? Melbourne: Orygen Youth Health Research Centre (2009). P.2 Available at: https://web.archive.org/web/20130428063353/http://www.headspace.org.au/core/Handlers/MediaHandler.ashx?mediaId=4896 (Accessed 18 March 2019).

101   Hetrick S. Parker A. Purcell R. Evidence Summary: Using SSRI Antidepressants and Other Newer Antidepressants to Treat Depression in Young People: What are the issues and what is the evidence? Melbourne: Headspace, National Youth Mental Health Foundation (2015). Available at: https://headspace.org.au/assets/Uploads/Resource-library/Health-professionals/ssri-v2-pdf.pdf (Accessed 20 November 2019).

102   Hetrick S, Purcell R. Evidence Summary: Using SSRI Antidepressants to Treat Depression in Young People: What are the Issues and What is the Evidence? Melbourne: Orygen Youth Health Research Centre (2009). P. 2 https://web.archive.org/web/20130428063353/http://www.headspace.org.au/core/Handlers/MediaHandler.ashx?mediaId=4896 (accessed 18 March 2019).

103   Hetrick S, Purcell R. Evidence Summary: Using SSRI Antidepressants to Treat Depression in Young People: What are the Issues and What is the Evidence? Melbourne: Orygen Youth Health Research Centre (2009). P. 2 https://web.archive.org/web/20130428063353/http://www.headspace.org.au/core/Handlers/MediaHandler.ashx?mediaId=4896 (accessed 18 March 2019).

104   Jill Stark. Youth mental health team too free with drugs: audit, The Age. July 8, 2012 https://www.theage.com.au/national/youth-mental-health-team-too-free-with-drugs-audit-20120707-21o29.html (accessed 4 June 2020).

105   Hetrick SE, Thompson A, Yuen K, Finch S, Parker AG. Is there a gap between recommended and 'real world' practice in the management of depression in young people? A medical file audit of practice. BMC Health Serv Res. 2012;12:178. Published 2012 Jun 27. doi:10.1186/1472-6963-12-178 https://www.ncbi.nlm.nih.gov/pmc/articles/PMC3444314/ (accessed 4 June 2020).

106   Sarah Hetrick, Rosemary Purcell, Patrick McGorry, Alison Yung, Andrew Chanen, (2009) Evidence Summary: Using SSRI Antidepressants to Treat Depression in Young People: What are the Issues and What is the Evidence? Headspace, Evidence Summary Writers 2009 Orygen Youth Health Research Centre Previously available at http://www.headspace.org.au/core/Handlers/MediaHandler.ashx?mediaId=4896 See https://web.archive.org/web/20130428063353/http://www.headspace.org.au/core/Handlers/MediaHandler.ashx?mediaId=4896 (accessed 18 March 2019).

107   Orygen Youth Health. Medications for Depression. Melbourne: Orygen (2009).https://oyh.org.au/sites/oyh.org.au/files/factsheets/oyh_fs_depmeds.pdf (accessed 18 November 2019).

108   Margot J. Suicide prevention experts may have got it 'horribly wrong'. Australian Financial Review. June 9 2020 https://www.afr.com/policy/health-and-education/suicide-prevention-experts-may-have-got-it-horribly-wrong-20200606-p5506d (accessed 15 July 2020).

109   McCauley D. Health Minister orders review after study links antidepressants and youth suicide. The Sydney Morning Herald. 14 June 2020 https://www.smh.com.au/politics/federal/health-minister-orders-review-after-study-links-antidepressants-and-youth-suicide-20200609-p550yr.html (accessed 15 July 2020).

110   Whitely M. Raven M. Jureidini J. Antidepressant Prescribing and Suicide/Self-Harm by Young Australians: Regulatory Warnings, Contradictory Advice, and Long-Term Trends. Frontiers in Psychiatry. June 2020 https://www.frontiersin.org/article/10.3389/fpsyt.2020.00478 (accessed 15 July 2020).

111   Hickie I. Curriculum Vitae: Ian Hickie AM MD FRANZCP FASSA. Available at: http://api.profiles.sydney.edu.au/AcademicProfiles/profile/resource?urlid=ian.hickie&type=cv (accessed 18 November 2019).

112   Hall WD, Mant A, Mitchell PB, Rendle VA, Hickie IB, McManus P. Association between antidepressant prescribing and suicide in Australia, 1991-2000: trend analysis. BMJ (2003) 326:1008. doi: https://www.bmj.com/content/326/7397/1008 (accessed 4 June 2020).

113   Sebastian Rosenberg, Ian Hickie. No gold medals: Assessing Australia's international mental health performance Australasian Psychiatry. 8 October 2018 https://journals.sagepub.com/doi/10.1177/1039856218804335 (accessed 12 August 2020).

114   Hickie I, Scott E. Understanding depression. Camperdown NSW: Educational Health Solutions and Brain & Mind Research Institute. Available at: https://web.archive.org/web/20091015092847/http://www.bmri.org.au/docs/understandingdepression.pdf (accessed 19 November 2019).

115   Hickie I. (2007) Is depression overdiagnosed? No. BMJ (2007) 335(7615):329. doi: 10.1136/

bmj.39268.497350.AD https://www.ncbi.nlm.nih.gov/pmc/articles/PMC1949449/ (accessed 4 June 2020).

116   Hickie I. (2007) Is depression overdiagnosed? No. BMJ (2007) 335(7615):329. doi: 10.1136/bmj.39268.497350.AD https://www.ncbi.nlm.nih.gov/pmc/articles/PMC1949449/ (accessed 4 June 2020).

117   Fora TV. Is Depression Being Over-Diagnosed? – Ian Hickie and Tanveer Ahmed [televised debate] (May 17, 2010). https://www.youtube.com/watch?v=qd6-Y8OYkX4 (accessed 18 November 2019).

118   Hickie IB, McGorry PD. Guidelines for youth depression: time to incorporate new perspectives. MJA (August 2010) 193(3):133-4. https://www.mja.com.au/journal/2010/193/3/guidelines-youth-depression-time-incorporate-new-perspectives (accessed 4 June 2020).

119   Gibbons RD, Brown CH, Hur K, Marcus SM, Bhaumik DK, Erkens JA, et al. Early evidence on the effects of regulators' suicidality warnings on SSRI prescriptions and suicide in children and adolescents. Am J Psychiatry (2007) https://ajp.psychiatryonline.org/doi/full/10.1176/appi.ajp.2007.07030454 (accessed 15 July 2020).

120   Hickie IB, McGorry PD. Guidelines for youth depression: time to incorporate new perspectives. MJA (August 2010) 193(3):133-4. https://www.mja.com.au/journal/2010/193/3/guidelines-youth-depression-time-incorporate-new-perspectives (accessed 4 June 2020).

121   Gibbons RD, Hur K, Bhaumik DK, Mann J. The relationship between antidepressant prescription rates and rate of early adolescent suicide. American Journal of Psychiatry (2006) 163:1898-1904. doi: 10.1176/ajp.2006.163.11.1898 https://ajp.psychiatryonline.org/doi/10.1176/ajp.2006.163.11.1898 (accessed 4 June 2006).

122   Jureidini J. The black box warning: Decreased prescriptions and increased youth suicide? American Journal of Psychiatry (2007) 164:1907. https://pubmed.ncbi.nlm.nih.gov/18056248/ (accessed 4 June 2020).

123   Hickie IB, McGorry PD. Guidelines for youth depression: time to incorporate new perspectives. MJA (August 2010) 193(3):133-4. https://www.mja.com.au/journal/2010/193/3/guidelines-youth-depression-time-incorporate-new-perspectives (accessed 4 June 2020).

124   Simon GE, Savarino J, Operskalski B, Wang PS. Suicide risk during antidepressant treatment. Am J Psychiatry (2006) 163:41-7. https://pubmed.ncbi.nlm.nih.gov/16390887/ (accessed 4 June 2020)

125   Hickie IB, McGorry PD. Guidelines for youth depression: time to incorporate new perspectives. MJA (August 2010) 193(3):133-4. https://www.mja.com.au/journal/2010/193/3/guidelines-youth-depression-time-incorporate-new-perspectives (accessed 4 June 2020).

126   Adverse Drug Reactions Advisory Committee (Therapeutic Goods Administration). Suicidality with SSRIs: adults and children. Australian Adverse Drug Reactions Bulletin (August 2005) 24(5). P. 14 Available at: https://www.tga.gov.au/publication-issue/australian-adverse-drug-reactions-bulletin-vol-24-no-4#a1 (Accessed 19 November 2019).

127   Hall WD, Mant A, Mitchell PB, Rendle VA, Hickie IB, McManus P. Association between antidepressant prescribing and suicide in Australia, 1991-2000: trend analysis. BMJ (2003) p. 32 326:1008. doi: https://doi.org/10.1136/bmj.326.7397.1008 (accessed 4 June 2020).

128   Adverse Drug Reactions Advisory Committee (Therapeutic Goods Administration). Suicidality with SSRIs: adults and children. Australian Adverse Drug Reactions Bulletin (August 2005) 24(5). P. 14 Available at: https://www.tga.gov.au/publication-issue/australian-adverse-drug-reactions-bulletin-vol-24-no-4#a1 (Accessed 19 November 2019).

129   Therapeutic Goods Administration. Antidepressants — communicating risks and benefits to patients. Medicines Safety Update). (October-December 2016) 7(5). Available at: https://www.tga.gov.au/publication-issue/medicines-safety-update-volume-7-number-5-october-december-2016#a2 (accessed 11 April 2019).

130   Australian Institute of Health and Welfare. Mental health services—in brief 2016. Cat. no. HSE 180. Canberra: AIHW (2016). (pp. 24-25) https://www.aihw.gov.au/getmedia/681f0689-8360-4116-b1cc-9d2276b65703/20299.pdf.aspx?inline=true (accessed 13 August 2018).

131   See Specialist in Life campaign for GPs Website at https://www.myhealthcareer.com.au/medicine/medicine-specialist-in-life-campaign/ (accessed 15 July 2020).

132   Irving G, Neves AL, Dambha-Miller H, et al. International variations in primary care physician consultation time: a systematic review of 67 countries. BMJ Open 2017;7:e017902. doi:10.1136/bmjopen-2017-017902 https://bmjopen.bmj.com/content/7/10/e017902 (accessed 4 June 2020).

133   "For an 'average' 100 GP-patient encounters, GPs provided 102 medications and 39 clinical

treatments (such as advice and counselling), undertook 18 procedures, made 10 referrals to medical specialists and 6 to allied health services, and placed 48 pathology test orders and 11 imaging test orders (Table 5.1)." Britt H, Miller GC, Henderson J, Bayram C, Harrison C, Valenti L, Pan Y, Charles J, Pollack AJ, Wong C, Gordon J. General practice activity in Australia 2015–16. General practice series no. 40. Sydney: Sydney University Press, 2016, p.34 file:///C:/Users/177421E/Downloads/9781743325148_ONLINE%20(2).pdf (accessed 4 June 2020).

134   ABC Radio 720 Perth. Breakfast with Nadia Mitsopolous. 24 April 2019. Interviews with Dr Martin Whitely, PsychWatch Australia, and Dr Harry Nespolon, President Royal Australian College of General Practitioners.

135   Whitely M. Massive media coverage of PsychWatch Australia's blog revealing 1 in 8 Aussies take antidepressants. PsychWatch Australia website 2019. Available at https://www.psychwatchaustralia.com/post/massive-media-coverage-of-psychwatch-australia-s-blog-revealing-1-in-8-aussies-take-antidepressants (accessed 14 April 2020).

136   Harvey C, Videnieks M. The new abuse excuse. The Australian. May 25, 2001, p. 14.

137   Gregory E. Simon and Michael VonKorff, Suicide Mortality among Patients Treated for Depression in an Insured Population American Journal of Epidemiology 1998 Vol. 147, No. 2. Available at https://pdfs.semanticscholar.org/65e8/c5a4298167106fea861b7bc4c9ff76cab304.pdf (accessed 29 June 2020).

138   A detailed analysis and refutation of previous similar '1 in 6' claims is available on pages 147-155 of the PhD thesis 'Depression and antidepressants in Australia and beyond — a critical public health analysis' of Dr Melissa Raven. https://ro.uow.edu.au/cgi/viewcontent.cgi?article=4688&context=theses (accessed 29 June 2020).

139   Raven, M. (2012). Depression and antidepressants in Australia and beyond: A critical public health analysis. [dissertation/PhD thesis (pp. 147-155). University of Wollongong. http://ro.uow.edu.au/theses/3686/

140   Simon GE, VonKorff M. Suicide mortality among patients treated for depression in an insured population. American Journal of Epidemiology (1998)147(2):155-60. p. 155. https://academic.oup.com/aje/article/147/2/155/183271 (accessed 4 June 2020).

141   Hickie I. (2007) Is depression overdiagnosed? No. BMJ (2007) 335(7615):329. doi: 10.1136/bmj.39268.497350.AD https://www.ncbi.nlm.nih.gov/pmc/articles/PMC1949449/ (accessed 4 June 2020).

142   Robinson J, Bailey E, Browne V, Cox G, Hooper C. Raising the bar for youth suicide prevention. Melbourne: Orygen, The National Centre of Excellence in Youth Mental Health. (2016). Available at: https://www.orygen.org.au/Policy-Advocacy/Policy-Reports/Raising-the-bar-for-youth-suicide-prevention/orygen-Suicide-Prevention-Policy-Report.aspx?ext= (accessed 14 September 2019).

143   Karanges EA, Stephenson CP, McGregor IS. Longitudinal trends in the dispensing of psychotropic medications in Australia from 2009-2012: focus on children, adolescents and prescriber specialty. Australian and New Zealand Journal of Psychiatry (2014) 48(10):917-31. doi: 10.1177/0004867414538675 p. 28 https://journals.sagepub.com/doi/10.1177/0004867414538675 (accessed 4 June 2020).

144   Cairns R, Karanges EA, Wong A, Brown JA, Robinson J, Pearson S-A et al. (2019) Trends in self-poisoning and psychotropic drug use in people aged 5-19 years: a population-based retrospective cohort study in Australia. BMJ Open. 2019;9:e026001. doi: 10.1136/bmjopen-2018-026001 https://bmjopen.bmj.com/content/9/2/e026001 (accessed 4 June 2020).

145   Australian Research Alliance for Children & Youth. Report Card 2018: The Wellbeing of Young Australians. (2018). Available at: https://www.aracy.org.au/publications-resources/command/download_file/id/361/filename/ARACY_Report_Card_2018.pdf (accessed 15 March 2019).

146   Cairns R, Karanges EA, Wong A, Brown JA, Robinson J, Pearson S-A et al. (2019) Trends in self-poisoning and psychotropic drug use in people aged 5-19 years: a population-based retrospective cohort study in Australia. BMJ Open. 2019;9:e026001. doi: 10.1136/bmjopen-2018-026001 https://bmjopen.bmj.com/content/9/2/e026001 (accessed 4 June 2020).

147   Whitely M. Raven M. More young Australians suicide/self-harm and use antidepressants while experts dismiss FDA warning. PsychWatch Australia website. 1 June 2019 https://www.psychwatchaustralia.com/post/more-young-australians-suicide-self-harm-and-use-antidepressants-while-experts-dismiss-fda-warning (accessed 16 July 2020).

148   Whitely M. Raven M. More young Australians suicide/self-harm and use antidepressants

while experts dismiss FDA warning. PsychWatch Australia website. 1 June 2019 https://www.psychwatchaustralia.com/post/more-young-australians-suicide-self-harm-and-use-antidepressants-while-experts-dismiss-fda-warning (accessed 16 July 2020).
149   Whitely M. Raven M. Jureidini J. Antidepressant Prescribing and Suicide/Self-Harm by Young Australians: Regulatory Warnings, Contradictory Advice, and Long-Term Trends. Frontiers in Psychiatry. June 2020 https://www.frontiersin.org/article/10.3389/fpsyt.2020.00478 (accessed 15 July 2020).
150   Isacsson G, Rich CL, Jureidini J, Raven M. The increased use of antidepressants has contributed to the worldwide reduction in suicide rates. (Debate piece - Against) British Journal of Psychiatry (2010) https://www.researchgate.net/publication/44640948_The_increased_use_of_antidepressants_has_contributed_to_the_worldwide_reduction_in_suicide_rates (accessed 11 February 2019).
151   Whitely M. Hansard Western Australian Parliament [Wednesday, 25 May 2011] pp. 3984d-3994a. Perth, WA, Australia: Parliament of Western Australian (2011). http://www.parliament.wa.gov.au/Hansard/hansard.nsf/0/75032653ddacbe7f482578b100299ab4/$FILE/A38+S1+20110525+p3984d-3994a.pdf (accessed 16 July 2020).
152   Beyond Blue. Anxiety and depression: An information booklet. Melbourne: beyondblue. Hawthorn, VIC, Australia 2015 http://resources.beyondblue.org.au/prism/file?token=BL/0885 (accessed 17 November 2019).
153   Whitely M. Raven M. Jureidini J. Antidepressant Prescribing and Suicide/Self-Harm by Young Australians: Regulatory Warnings, Contradictory Advice, and Long-Term Trends. Frontiers in Psychiatry. June 2020 https://www.frontiersin.org/article/10.3389/fpsyt.2020.00478 (accessed 15 July 2020).
154   Hagan K. GetUp! calls for urgent reform to mental health policy. The Age (July 29, 2010) Available at: https://www.theage.com.au/national/victoria/getup-calls-for-urgent-reform-to-mental-health-policy-20100728-10w74.html (Accessed 11 April 2019).
155   Whitely M (2011) Hansard Western Australian Parliament [Wednesday, 25 May 2011] p3984d - 3994a. (pp. 3-8) Available at: http://www.parliament.wa.gov.au/Hansard/hansard.nsf/0/75032653ddacbe7f482578b100299ab4/$FILE/A38+S1+20110525+p3984d-3994a.pdf (accessed 11 February 2019).
156   Whitely M. Raven M. Jureidini J. Antidepressant Prescribing and Suicide/Self-Harm by Young Australians: Regulatory Warnings, Contradictory Advice, and Long-Term Trends. Frontiers in Psychiatry. June 2020 https://www.frontiersin.org/article/10.3389/fpsyt.2020.00478 (accessed 15 July 2020).
157   Whitely M. Raven M. Jureidini J. Antidepressant Prescribing and Suicide/Self-Harm by Young Australians: Regulatory Warnings, Contradictory Advice, and Long-Term Trends. Frontiers in Psychiatry. June 2020 https://www.frontiersin.org/article/10.3389/fpsyt.2020.00478 (accessed 15 July 2020).
158   Robinson J, Bailey E, Browne V, Cox G, Hooper C. Raising the bar for youth suicide prevention. Melbourne: Orygen, The National Centre of Excellence in Youth Mental Health. (2016). Available at: https://www.orygen.org.au/Policy-Advocacy/Policy-Reports/Raising-the-bar-for-youth-suicide-prevention/orygen-Suicide-Prevention-Policy-Report.aspx?ext= (Accessed 14 September 2019).
159   Robinson J, Bailey E, Browne V, Cox G, Hooper C. Raising the bar for youth suicide prevention. Melbourne: Orygen, The National Centre of Excellence in Youth Mental Health. (2016) p. 7 Av https://www.orygen.org.au/Policy/Policy-Reports/Raising-the-bar-for-youth-suicide-prevention/orygen-Suicide-Prevention-Policy-Report?ext (Accessed 14 September 2019).
160   Cairns R, Karanges EA, Wong A, Brown JA, Robinson J, Pearson S-A et al. (2019) Trends in self-poisoning and psychotropic drug use in people aged 5-19 years: a population-based retrospective cohort study in Australia. BMJ Open. 2019;9:e026001. doi: 10.1136/bmjopen-2018-026001 p. 4+6 https://bmjopen.bmj.com/content/9/2/e026001 (accessed 4 June 2020).
161   Karanges EA, Stephenson CP, McGregor IS. Longitudinal trends in the dispensing of psychotropic medications in Australia from 2009-2012: focus on children, adolescents and prescriber specialty. Australian and New Zealand Journal of Psychiatry (2014) 48(10):917-31. doi: 10.1177/0004867414538675 p. 28 https://journals.sagepub.com/doi/10.1177/0004867414538675 (accessed 4 June 2020).
162   Davey M. 'Struggling to cope': child suicide rates may rise as intentional self-poisoning rates double, Guardian Australia. 21 February 2019. Available at: https://www.theguardian.com/australia-news/2019/feb/21/struggling-to-cope-child-suicide-rates-may-rise-as-intentional-self-poisoning-rates-double (accessed 17 November 2019).

163   Ison S. It's time to rethink kids pills. *The West Australian*. 27 June 2019. Available at http://
enewspaper2.smedia.com.au/wandally/shared/ShowArticle.
aspx?doc=WAN%2F2019%2F06%2F27&entity=Ar01104&sk=A415DC25&f-
bclid=IwAR3PYvVtboWfBL6SfewRk65LlSicNEnVzJgYN_veQ06s_Ilxv6TA8e8-qMU (accessed 20
July 2019).

164   Whitely M. Letter to Prime Minister Scott Morison dated 24 June 2017 copy available at https://
www.psychwatchaustralia.com/post/dear-pm-re-youth-suicide-and-antidepressants-please-don-t-lis-
ten-to-the-same-failed-local-experts (accessed 20 July 2019).

165   Hengartner M.P. Plöderl M. Newer-Generation Antidepressants and Suicide Risk in
Randomized Controlled Trials: A Re-Analysis of the FDA Database. *Psychotherapy Psychosomatics*. 24
June 2019. https://www.karger.com/Article/Pdf/501215 (accessed 17 July 2019).

166   Whitely M. Raven M. Jureidini J. Antidepressant Prescribing and Suicide/Self-Harm by Young
Australians: Regulatory Warnings, Contradictory Advice, and Long-Term Trends. *Frontiers in Psychiatry*.
June 2020 https://www.frontiersin.org/article/10.3389/fpsyt.2020.00478 (accessed 15 July 2020).

167   Margot J. Suicide prevention experts may have got it 'horribly wrong'. Australian Financial
Review. June 9 2020 https://www.afr.com/policy/health-and-education/suicide-prevention-experts-
may-have-got-it-horribly-wrong-20200606-p5506d (accessed 15 July 2020).

168   ABC Radio National Drive with Patricia Karvelas Friday 12 June 2020 The interview begins
at the 27 minute 10 second mark of the podcast available at https://www.abc.net.au/radionational/
programs/drive/pm-issues-ultimatum-on-borders-indigenous-referendum-unlikely/12336770
(accessed 17 July 2020).

169   McCauley D. Health Minister orders review after study links antidepressants and youth suicide.
The Sydney Morning Herald. 14 June 2020 https://www.smh.com.au/politics/federal/health-minister-
orders-review-after-study-links-antidepressants-and-youth-suicide-20200609-p550yr.html (accessed
15 July 2020).

170   Julian Hill MHR Member for Bruce. Private Members' Business Hansard Federation Chamber 10
June 2020 https://www.aph.gov.au/Parliamentary_Business/Hansard/Hansard_Display?bid=chamber/
hansardr/5a20f627-6fba-4392-b834-9b1bc518612a/&sid=0252 (accessed 15 July 2020).

171   Lanai Scarr. 5yo kids in Anxiety Centres, *The West Australian* 5 June 2019 https://www.
pressreader.com/australia/the-west-australian/20190605/page/3/textview (accessed 15 July 2020).

172   Liberal Party of Australia, (2019) 'Our Plan for youth mental health and suicide prevention'
Available at https://www.liberal.org.au/our-plan-youth-mental-health-and-suicide-prevention
(accessed 28 May 2019).

173   Liberal Party of Australia, (2019) 'Our Plan for youth mental health and suicide prevention'
Available at https://www.liberal.org.au/our-plan-youth-mental-health-and-suicide-prevention
(accessed 28 May 2019).

174   Letter from Health Minister Greg Hunt to Dr Martin Whitely Editor/Publisher PsychWatch
Australia 1 August 2019 Full copy available at https://www.psychwatchaustralia.com/post/dear-pm-
re-youth-suicide-and-antidepressants-please-don-t-listen-to-the-same-failed-local-experts (accessed
12 June 2020).

175   Letter from Health Minister Greg Hunt to Dr Martin Whitely Editor/Publisher PsychWatch
Australia 1 August 2019 Full copy available at https://www.psychwatchaustralia.com/post/dear-pm-
re-youth-suicide-and-antidepressants-please-don-t-listen-to-the-same-failed-local-experts (accessed
12 June 2020).

176   The University of Melbourne Website. Find an Expert – Professor Patrick McGorry https://
findanexpert.unimelb.edu.au/profile/14906-patrick-mcgorry (accessed 30 June 2020).

177   Early Intervention in Psychiatry Website https://onlinelibrary.wiley.com/page/
journal/17517893/homepage/editorialboard.html (accessed 30 June 2020).

178   headspace website. About headspace Board https://headspace.org.au/about-us/the-headspace-
board/ (accessed 30 June 2020).

179   McGorry P. "A Stitch in Time" ... The Scope for Preventive Strategies in Early Psychosis.
European Archives in Psychiatry Clinical Neuroscience. 1998 https://www.ncbi.nlm.nih.gov/
pubmed/9561350 (accessed 5 June 2020)..

180   Alison R. Yung and Patrick D. McGorry, The Prodromal Phase of First-Episode Psychosis: Past

and Current Conceptualizations Article in Schizophrenia Bulletin· February 1996. Available at https://www.ncbi.nlm.nih.gov/pubmed/8782291 (Accessed 17 May 2020).

181   Professor David Castle, Is it appropriate to treat people at high-risk of psychosis before first onset — No, *Medical Journal of Australia*. 21 May 2012. https://www.mja.com.au/journal/2012/196/9/it-appropriate-treat-people-high-risk-psychosis-first-onset-no (accessed 5 June 2020)..

182   Evidence Summary: Identification of young people at risk of developing psychosis headspace National Youth Mental Health Foundation, 2015.p. 4 https://headspace.org.au/assets/download-cards/Evidence-Summary-Identification-of-Young-People-at-Risk-Developing-Psychosis.pdf (accessed 5 June 2020).

183   Evidence Summary: Identification of young people at risk of developing psychosis headspace National Youth Mental Health Foundation, 2015.p. 2 https://headspace.org.au/assets/download-cards/Evidence-Summary-Identification-of-Young-People-at-Risk-Developing-Psychosis.pdf (accessed 5 June 2020).

184   Patrick D. McGorry, Lisa J. Phillips, Alison R. Yung, Early Intervention in Psychotic Disorders pp 101-122 Recognition and Treatment of the Pre-psychotic Phase of Psychotic Disorders Frontier or Fantasy? https://link.springer.com/chapter/10.1007/978-94-010-0892-1_5 (accessed 5 June 2020).

185   Professor David Castle, Is it appropriate to treat people at high-risk of psychosis before first onset — No. Medical Journal of Australia. 21 May 2012 https://www.mja.com.au/journal/2012/196/9/it-appropriate-treat-people-high-risk-psychosis-first-onset-no (accessed 5 June 2020)..

186   Professor McGorry said. Transdiagnostic Psychiatry – The new frontier? Orygen Website 16 October 2019. https://www.orygen.org.au/About/News-And-Events/2019/Transdiagnostic-psychiatry-the-new-frontier (accessed 12 June 2020).

187   Frances A. Australia's Reckless Experiment In Early Intervention – prevention that will do more harm than good. *Psychology Today*. May 31 2011 http://www.psychologytoday.com/blog/dsm5-in-distress/201105/australias-reckless-experiment-in-early-intervention (accessed 12 June 2020).

188   Frances, A. (2010) DSM5 'Psychosis risk syndrome'—Far too risky, *Psychology Today* Posted Mar 18, 2010 http://www.psychologytoday.com/blog/dsm5-in-distress/201003/dsm5-psychosis-risk-syndrome-far-too-risky (accessed 12 June 2020).

189   Lisa Pryor, Minds at risk, *The Monthly*, July 2011 https://www.themonthly.com.au/issue/2011/june/1314794127/lisa-pryor/minds-risk (accessed 12 June 2020).

190   Amy Maxem, Psychosis risk syndrome excluded from DSM-5, Nature, 9 May 2012. https://www.nature.com/news/psychosis-risk-syndrome-excluded-from-dsm-5-1.10610 (accessed 12 June 2020).

191   McGorry P. DSMV 'risk syndrome': a good start, should go further, Psychiatry Update. Previously available at http://www.psychiatryupdate.com.au/news/DSM-V-risk-syndrome-a-good-start-should-go-further (accessed 28 May 2011).

192   McGorry, P.D. Risk Syndromes, clinical staging and DSM V; New diagnostic infrastructure for early intervention in psychiatry, Schizophrenia Research. 2010 http://www.ecnp-congress.eu/~/media/Files/ecnp/communication/talk-of-the-month/mcgorry/McGorry%20RIsk%20Syndrome%202010.pdf (accessed 13 June 2020).

193   The World Today – Professor McGorry hits back at critics, 20 May 2011 www.abc.net.au/worldtoday/content/2011/s3222359.htm (accessed 13 June 2020).

194   Lisa Pryor, Minds at risk, *The Monthly*, July 2011 https://www.themonthly.com.au/issue/2011/june/1314794127/lisa-pryor/minds-risk (accessed 12 June 2020).

195   Amy Corderoy, About-turn on treatment of the Young, *Sydney Morning Herald*, February 20, 2012 http://www.smh.com.au/national/health/aboutturn-on-treatment-of-the-young-20120219-1th8a.html (accessed 13 June 2020).

196   Previously available at http://www.speedupsitstill.com/patrick_mcgorry_deserves_praise_about_turn_psychosis_risk_disorder/index.html..

197   McGorry PD, Hickie IB, Yung AR, Pantelis C, Jackson HJ, Clinical staging of psychiatric disorders: a heuristic framework for choosing earlier, safer and more effective interventions. *Australia New Zealand Journal of Psychiatry* https://www.ncbi.nlm.nih.gov/pubmed/16866756.

198   Yung, A.R. & McGorry, P. (2007) Prediction of psychosis: setting the stage, *British Journal of Psychiatry*, 2007. http://bjp.rcpsych.org/cgi/content/full/191/51/s1 (accessed 7 December 2010).

199   Mrazek, P. J. & Haggerty, R. J. (eds) Reducing Reducing Risks for Mental Disorders: Frontiers

for Preventive Risks for Mental Disorders: Frontiers for Preventive Intervention research. National Academy Press. . National Academy Press 1994..

200   Yung, A.R. & McGorry, P. (2007) Prediction of psychosis: setting the stage, *British Journal of Psychiatry*, 2007. http://bjp.rcpsych.org/cgi/content/full/191/51/s1 (accessed 7 December 2010).

201   McGorry P.D. Is early intervention in the major psychiatric disorders justified? Yes, BMJ, 337:a695 2008. http://www.bmj.com/cgi/content/full/337/aug04_1/a695 (accessed 3 August 2010) .

202   Previously available at http://speedupsitstill.com/reply-patrick-mcgorry-early-intervention-psychosis#more-1075.

203   Previously available at http://speedupsitstill.com/reply-patrick-mcgorry-early-intervention-psychosis.

204   Stark, J. Drug trial scrapped amid outcry. *The Age*. 21 August 2011 http://www.theage.com.au/national/drug-trial-scrapped-amid-outcry-20110820-1j3vy.html (accessed 13 June 2020).

205   Stark, J. Drug trial scrapped amid outcry. *The Age*. 21 August 2011 http://www.theage.com.au/national/drug-trial-scrapped-amid-outcry-20110820-1j3vy.html (accessed 13 June 2020).

206   TianHong Zhang et al., Real-world effectiveness of antipsychotic treatment in psychosis prevention in a 3-year cohort of 517 individuals at clinical high risk from the SHARP (ShangHai At Risk for Psychosis). *Australian and New Zealand Journal of Psychiatry*. May 2020. https://journals.sagepub.com/doi/full/10.1177/0004867420917449 (accessed 15 August 2020).

207   Orygen website. $33 Million grant for psychosis research sets Australian record for medical research funding. 16 September 2020. https://www.orygen.org.au/About/News-And-Events/2020/$33-million-grant-for-psychosis-research-sets-Aust.

208   Orygen website. $33 Million grant for psychosis research sets Australian record for medical research funding. 16 September 2020. https://www.orygen.org.au/About/News-And-Events/2020/$33-million-grant-for-psychosis-research-sets-Aust.

209   National Institute of Health website. Accelerating Medicines Partnership – Schizophrenia page. https://www.nih.gov/research-training/accelerating-medicines-partnership-amp/schizophrenia (accessed 26 September 2020).

210   Accelerating Medicines Partnership [Schizophrenia Research] partners include Boehringer Ingelheim Pharmaceuticals, Inc.; Janssen Research & Development,; Otsuka Pharmaceutical Development & Commercialization, Inc. The Partnership steering committee includes representatives from each partner organizations and will provide detailed technical analyses of key scientific, policy, or informatics issues that arise during implementation.' National Institute of Health website. Project Information page: *Trajectories and Predictors in the Clinical High Risk for Psychosis population: Australian Network of Clinics and international Partners* https://projectreporter.nih.gov/project_info_description.cfm?aid=10092863&icde=51660550&ddparam=&ddvalue=&ddsub=&cr=1&csb=default&cs=ASC&pball= (Accessed 30 September 2020).

211   Fran Kelly interview with Professor Patrick McGorry. Youth mental health researchers awarded $33 million from US institute ABC Radio RN Breakfast. 16 September 2020. https://www.abc.net.au/radionational/programs/breakfast/youth-mental-health-researchers-awarded/12668472#:~:text=Youth%20mental%20health%20researchers%20awarded%20%2433%20million%20from%20US%20institute,-On%20RN%20Breakfast&text=The%20Australian%20youth%20mental%20health,Health%20in%20the%20United%20States .

212   Fran Kelly interview with Professor Patrick McGorry. Youth mental health researchers awarded $33 million from US institute ABC Radio RN Breakfast. 16 September 2020. https://www.abc.net.au/radionational/programs/breakfast/youth-mental-health-researchers-awarded/12668472#:~:text=Youth%20mental%20health%20researchers%20awarded%20%2433%20million%20from%20US%20institute,-On%20RN%20Breakfast&text=The%20Australian%20youth%20mental%20health,Health%20in%20the%20United%20States.

213   Orygen website. $33 Million grant for psychosis research sets Australian record for medical research funding. 16 September 2020. https://www.orygen.org.au/About/News-And-Events/2020/$33-million-grant-for-psychosis-research-sets-Aust.

214   Fran Kelly interview with Professor Patrick McGorry. Youth mental health researchers awarded $33 million from US institute ABC Radio RN Breakfast. 16 September 2020. https://www.abc.net.au/radionational/programs/breakfast/youth-mental-health-researchers-

awarded/12668472#:~:text=Youth%20mental%20health%20researchers%20awarded%20%2433%20
million%20from%20US%20institute,-On%20RN%20Breakfast&text=The%20Australian%20
youth%20mental%20health,Health%20in%20the%20United%20States.

215   Orygen — The National Centre for Excellence in Youth Mental Health, National reform and
the roll-out of EPPIC. 18 October 2018 https://www.orygen.org.au/About/News-And-Events/2018/
roll-out-of-EPPIC (accessed 2 September 2019).

216   Patrick D McGorry, Chris Tanti, Ryan Stokes, Ian B Hickie, Kate Carnell, Lyndel K Littlefield
and John Moran. *headspace: Australia's National Youth Mental Health Foundation — where
young minds come first. Medical Journal of Australia* 1 October 2007 https://www.mja.com.au/
journal/2007/187/7/headspace-australias-national-youth-mental-health-foundation-where-young-
minds (accessed 12 June 2019).

217   headspace webpage. headspace early psychosis. https://headspace.org.au/our-services/
earlypsychosis/headspace-early-psychosis/ (accessed 12 June 2019).

218   headspace webpage. Welcome to headspace services. https://headspace.org.au/welcome-to-
headspace-centres/ (accessed 12 June 2019).

219   Australian of the year awards, Australian of the year announced. 25 January 2010 https://
www.australianoftheyear.org.au/news-and-media/tour-of-honour-2013/news-and-media/news/arti-
cle/?id=australians-of-the-year-announced (accessed 12 June 2019).

220   Williams, D (18 June 2006) Drugs Before Diagnosis? *Time* http://www.time.com/time/
magazine/article/0,9171,1205408,00.html (accessed 18 November 2010).

221   McGorry P.D. 'Is early intervention in the major psychiatric disorders justified? Yes', BMJ
2008;337:a695 http://www.bmj.com/cgi/content/full/337/aug04_1/a695(accessed 3 August 2010).

222   International Early Psychosis Association. Parkville, VIC, Australia (2020). *Sponsors* https://
iepa.org.au/sponsors/ (Accessed 8 May 2020)..

223   Orygen Youth Health, Research Centre – Other Funding. http://rc.oyh.org.au/
ResearchCentreStructure/otherfunding (accessed 3 August 2010).

224   Address to the National Press Club Canberra by Prof. Patrick McGorry. 7 July 2010.

225   O'Neill, Luke, McGorry urges better access to mental health care. Irish Echo – Australia's Irish
Newspaper 15 March 2011..

226   Address to the National Press Club Canberra by Prof. Patrick McGorry. 7 July 2010 .

227   Prof Patrick McGorry. A 21st century Approach to Mental Health Care for Australia. 2010
Maurice Blackburn Oration https://www.moreland.vic.gov.au/globalassets/key-docs/speech/mau-
rice-blackburn-oration-2010--a-21st-century-approach-to-mental-health-care.pdf (accessed 12 June
2019).

228   *Insight* SBS television 27 July 2010 transcript available at https://www.sbs.com.au/news/sites/sbs.
com.au.news/files/transcripts/363445_insight_mentalhealth_transcript.html (accessed 12 June 2019).

229   Adjunct Professor Mendoza was co-author of the "Not for Service" report which was issued
in 2005. Apart from the Commonwealth Government, the report was funded by unrestricted grants
from AstraZeneca, Bristol-Myers Squibb, Eli Lilly Australia, GlaxoSmithKline, Medicines Australia,
Pfizer Australia and Wyeth. (Not For Service: Experiences of Injustice and Despair in Mental Health
Care in Australia, Mental Health Council of Australia, Canberra, 2005. http://www.hreoc.gov.au/
disability_rights/notforservice/documents/NFS_Finaldoc.pdf (3 August 2010). He is also a principal
of ConNetica Consulting Pty Ltd, which listed Eli Lilly as one of its private sector clients (ConNetica
Consulting, *About Us* http://connetica.com.au/about_us (accessed 3 August 2010).

230   ABC News. Roxon, Dutton trade blows in health debate. 11 August 2010 https://www.abc.net.
au/news/2010-08-11/roxon-dutton-trade-blows-in-health-debate/940908?site=news (accessed 12
June 2019).

231   Carr, Vaughan. Letter to the Editor, Mental health funding. *The Australian*. 10 July 2010. http://
www.theaustralian.com.au/news/opinion/mental-health-funding/story-fn558imw-1225890005936.

232   Carr V. Mentally ill of all ages need services. *The Australian*. 8 July 2010. http://
www.theaustralian.com.au/news/opinion/mentally-ill-of-all-ages-need-services/story-
e6frg6zo-1225889141003 (accessed 30 April 2011) .

233   Advisory Group to Guide Mental Health Reforms (23 December 2010), *Pro Bono News*
Advisory Group to Guide Mental Health Reforms (accessed 26 April 2011).

234 Advisory Group to Guide Mental Health Reforms, *Pro Bono News* Posted: Thursday, December 23, 2010 http://www.probonoaustralia.com.au/news/2010/12/advisory-group-guide-mental-health-reforms (accessed 26 April 2011).

235 Including, Connecting, Contributing- A Blueprint to Transform Mental Health and Social Participation in Australia March 2011 Prepared by the Independent Mental Health Reform Group, Monsignor David Cappo, Professor Patrick McGorry, Professor Ian Hickie, Sebastian Rosenberg John Moran, Matthew Hamilton http://sydney.edu.au/bmri/docs/260311-BLUEPRINT.pdf (accessed 26 April 2011).

236 Orygen Youth Health — Early Psychosis Prevention Intervention Centre website http://www.eppic.org.au/about-us (accessed 26 April 2011).

237 National Mental Health Reform Statement by Hon. Nicola Roxon Minister, Hon. Jenny Macklin and the Hon. Mark Butler 10 May 2011 Available at http://www.hpv.health.gov.au/internet/budget/publishing.nsf/Content/379A1A7327F54C2ACA257CA0003FF52B/$File/DHA%20Ministerial.PDF (accessed 1 September 2019).

238 NATIONAL MENTAL HEALTH REFORM 2011-12,Strengthening the focus on the mental health needs of children, families and youth Page last updated: 06 June 2011, Budget Measure: Additional Early Psychosis Prevention and Intervention Centres (EPPIC) - $222.4 million over the next five years. "A total of 16 EPPIC sites nationally will have the capacity to assist more than 11,000 young Australians with, or at risk of developing, psychotic mental illness; promoting an early and positive experience of managing mental illness and protecting them from poor education and employment outcomes, homelessness and other forms of disadvantage. https://www1.health.gov.au/internet/publications/publishing.nsf/Content/nmhr11-12~nmhr11-12-priorities~children (accessed 23 September 2019).

239 Bryan Littlely, Greg Kelton, Catherine Hockley, Catholic priest Monsignor David Cappo resigns as chair of Mental Health Commission, *The Advertiser.* 16 September 2011. https://www.adelaidenow.com.au/news/south-australia/act-on-claims-or-ill-go-public-xenophon/news-story/4039e01668d2dc95e031bf09fe1e5f8e (accessed 12 June 2019).

240 *Sue Dunlevy* 'Schism opens over ills of the mind' *The Australian. 16* June 2011. https://www.theaustralian.com.au/news/inquirer/schism-opens-over-ills-of-the-mind/news-story/7d9b-4717404ff875fd2b9747e17817d8 (accessed 13 June 2020).

241 *Sue Dunlevy* 'Schism opens over ills of the mind' *The Australian. 16* June 2011. https://www.theaustralian.com.au/news/inquirer/schism-opens-over-ills-of-the-mind/news-story/7d9b-4717404ff875fd2b9747e17817d8 (accessed 13 June 2020).

242 Previously available at http://www.eppic.org.au/about-us.

243 Previously available at http://cp.oyh.org.au/ClinicalPrograms/pace.

244 '1 Identification, monitoring and treatment for individuals with an 'at risk' mental state are optimal - All individuals with an 'at risk' mental state (e.g. siblings of EPPIC clients) will be referred to PACE Clinic* for assessment'. Previously available at http://www.eppic.org.au/sites/all/files/EPPICguidelines_web.pdf.

245 Extract from Hansard Thursday, 31 May 2012 p636b-639a Western Australian Legislative Assembly. http://www.parliament.wa.gov.au/Hansard/hansard.nsf/0/57de-02ae107600d148257a220046f171/$FILE/A38%20S1%2020120531%20p636b-639a.pdf (accessed 13 June 2020).

246 hYEPP (headspace Youth Early Psychosis Program) – Joondalup website https://www.health-direct.gov.au/australian-health-services/23023371/hyepp-headspace-youth-early-psychosis-program-joondalup/services/joondalup-6027-grand (accessed 13 June 2020).

247 headspace webpage. headspace early psychosis. https://headspace.org.au/our-services/earlypsychosis/headspace-early-psychosis/ (accessed 12 June 2020).

248 Orygen Youth Health Centre, 2009, "Comprehensive Assessment of At Risk Mental State (CAARMS) Training DVD", The PACE Clinic, Department of Psychiatry, University of Melbourne. Extract available at https://www.psychwatchaustralia.com/mcgorry-video-fails-commonsense-tes (accessed 3 September 2012).

249 Orygen Youth Health Centre, 2009, "Comprehensive Assessment of At Risk Mental State (CAARMS) Training DVD", The PACE Clinic, Department of Psychiatry, University of Melbourne. Extract available at https://www.psychwatchaustralia.com/mcgorry-video-fails-commonsense-tes (accessed 3 September 2012).

250   Whitely M, Jureidini J. Patrick McGorry's Orygen Youth Health 'Ultra High Risk of Psychosis' training video fails the common sense test - Watch and ask yourself: Is Nick Sick? originally posted on September 5, 2012 available at https://www.psychwatchaustralia.com/mcgorry-video-fails-commonsense-tes (accessed 3 September 2012).

251   Whitely M, Jureidini J. Patrick McGorry's Orygen Youth Health 'Ultra High Risk of Psychosis' training video fails the common sense test - Watch and ask yourself: Is Nick Sick? originally posted on September 5, 2012 available at https://www.psychwatchaustralia.com/mcgorry-video-fails-commonsense-tes (accessed 3 September 2012).

252   Whitely M, McLaren N. Patrick McGorry's Orygen Youth Health 'Ultra High Risk of Psychosis' training video fails the common sense test - Watch and ask yourself: Is Nick Sick? originally posted on September 5, 2012 available at https://www.psychwatchaustralia.com/mcgorry-video-fails-commonsense-tes (accessed 3 September 2012).

253   Amos A. Assessing the cost of early intervention in psychosis: a systematic review. *Australian New Zealand Journal of Psychiatry*. 2012 https://www.ncbi.nlm.nih.gov/pubmed/22696550.

254   McGorry P. et. al. Introduction to 'Early psychosis: a bridge to the future' *British Journal of Psychiatry* 2005. https://www.researchgate.net/profile/Merete_Nordentoft/publication/7689931_Introduction_to_%27Early_psychosis_A_bridge_to_the_future%27/links/57f7e18b08ae280dd0bcc950/Introduction-to-Early-psychosis-A-bridge-to-the-future.pdf (accessed 1 September 2019).

255   Stark, J. (2011, August 21). Drug trial scrapped amid outcry. *The Age*. http://www.theage.com.au/national/drug-trial-scrapped-amid-outcry-20110820-1j3vy.html .

256   Kathy McLiesh, Winding back early psychosis service short-sighted: Patrick McGorry 9 June 2016 https://www.abc.net.au/news/2016-06-09/move-to-wind-back-youth-early-psychosis-service-short-sighted/7495084 (accessed 13 June 2020).

257   Orygen, National reform and the Roll out of EPPIC webpage https://www.orygen.org.au/About/News-And-Events/2018/roll-out-of-EPPIC (accessed 13 June 2020).

258   https://www.orygen.org.au/About/News-And-Events/2018/roll-out-of-EPPIC..

259   Orygen, National reform and the Roll out of EPPIC webpage https://www.orygen.org.au/About/News-And-Events/2018/roll-out-of-EPPIC (accessed 13 June 2020).

260   Liberal Party of Australia, (2019) 'Our Plan for youth mental health and suicide prevention' Available at https://www.liberal.org.au/our-plan-youth-mental-health-and-suicide-prevention (accessed 28 May 2019).

261   Australian Government Productivity Commission Mental Health Inquiry Report 30 June 2020 Action 23.6 p.1163 https://www.pc.gov.au/inquiries/completed/mental-health/report .

262   Muir K, Powell A, Patulny R, Flaxman S, McDermott S, Oprea I, et al. Headspace Evaluation Report: Independent Evaluation of headspace: the National Youth Mental Health Foundation (SPRC Report 19/19). Sydney: Social Policy Research Centre (SPRC), UNSW, Australia; 2009. P. 125 Available at https://headspace.org.au/assets/Uploads/Corporate/Publications-and-research/final-independent-evaluation-of-headspace-report.pdf (accessed 6 June 2019).

263   Hilferty F, Cassells R, Muir K, Duncan A, Christensen D, Mitrou F, et al. Is headspace making a difference to young people's lives? Final Report of the independent evaluation of the headspace program. (SPRC Report 08/2015). Sydney: Social Policy Research Centre, UNSW, Australia; 2015. Available at https://headspace.org.au/assets/Uploads/Evaluation-of-headspace-program.pdf (accessed 6 June 2019).

264   https://www.abc.net.au/news/2019-04-28/headspace-failing-australias-youth-experts-say/11039776 .

265   Muir K, Powell A, Patulny R, Flaxman S, McDermott S, Oprea I, et al. Headspace Evaluation Report: Independent Evaluation of headspace: the National Youth Mental Health Foundation (SPRC Report 19/19). Sydney: Social Policy Research Centre (SPRC), UNSW, Australia; 2009. P. 125 Available at https://headspace.org.au/assets/Uploads/Corporate/Publications-and-research/final-independent-evaluation-of-headspace-report.pdf (accessed 6 June 2019).

266   Hilferty F, Cassells R, Muir K, Duncan A, Christensen D, Mitrou F, et al. Is headspace making a difference to young people's lives? Final Report of the independent evaluation of the headspace program. (SPRC Report 08/2015). Sydney: Social Policy Research Centre, UNSW, Australia; 2015. Available at https://headspace.org.au/assets/Uploads/Evaluation-of-headspace-program.pdf (accessed 6 June 2019).

267   Jorm AF. How effective are 'headspace' youth mental health services? *The Australian and New Zealand journal of psychiatry*. 2015,49(10).861-2. P. 862 https://minerva-access.unimelb.edu.au/bitstream/handle/11343/91134/how%20effective%20are.pdf?sequence=3&isAllowed=y (accessed 13 June 2020).

268   Looi JC, Allison S, Bastiampillai T Leviathans: Headspace-like behemoths swallow resources *Australian New Zealand Journal of Psychiatry*. 25 September 2019 https://www.ncbi.nlm.nih.gov/pubmed/31552751 (accessed 13 June 2020).

269   National Mental Health Commission, The National Review of Mental Health Programmes and Services. Sydney, NSW, Australia: 2014. vol. 2, p. 156 https://mhfa.com.au/sites/default/files/vol2-review-mh-programmes-services.pdf (accessed 13 June 2020).

270   National Mental Health Commission, The National Review of Mental Health Programmes and Services. Sydney, NSW, Australia: 2014 NMHC. vol. 1 p. 82.

271   Williams, D. Drugs Before Diagnosis? Time. 18 June 2006 http://www.time.com/time/magazine/article/0,9171,1205408,00.html (accessed 18 November 2010).

272   McGorry P. et al. Introduction to 'Early psychosis: a bridge to the future' *British Journal of Psychiatry* 2005. Available at https://www.researchgate.net/profile/Merete_Nordentoft/publication/7689931_Introduction_to_%27Early_psychosis_A_bridge_to_the_future%27/links/57f7e18b08ae280dd0bcc950/Introduction-to-Early-psychosis-A-bridge-to-the-future.pdf (accessed 1 September 2019).

273   McGorry P. et. al. Introduction to 'Early psychosis: a bridge to the future' *British Journal of Psychiatry* 2005. https://www.researchgate.net/profile/Merete_Nordentoft/publication/7689931_Introduction_to_%27Early_psychosis_A_bridge_to_the_future%27/links/57f7e18b08ae280dd0bcc950/Introduction-to-Early-psychosis-A-bridge-to-the-future.pdf (accessed 1 September 2019).

274   McGorry P. Opinion Piece, Mental health needs reform, not vague promises. *Herald Sun*. 4 November 2014 https://www.heraldsun.com.au/news/opinion/mental-health-needs-reform-not-vague-promises/news-story/8b122f66ea2c28d9e8e7ec566d2cf9bc (accessed 15 June 2020).

275   ABC (11 March 2010) Mental health system in crisis: McGorry, Lateline, Australian Broadcasting Corporation. Reporter: Tony Jones http://www.abc.net.au/lateline/content/2010/s2843609.htm (accessed 26 April 2011).

276   In a presentation on behalf of beyondblue, Professor Ian Hickie claimed the 12 month prevalence of mental disorders for Australia men is 17.4% and woman 18.0%. *Responding to the challenge of brain and mind disorders in Australia*, Ian Hickie MD FRANZCP Professor of Psychiatry, Brain and Mind Research Institute, University of Sydney& Clinical Advisor, beyondblue: the national depression initiative http://www.gptt.com.au/Exam%20preparation%20CK%20Khong/Mental%20Health/Depression%20adults%20hickie_slides.pdf.

277   *The Age* Julia Medew *August 9, 2010* McGorry Misleading the parliament http://www.theage.com.au/national/mcgorry-misleading-the-public-20100808-11qes.html.

278   Patrick McGorry defends early intervention on youth mental health, Croakey the Crikey Health Blog August 17, 2010. https://www.croakey.org/patrick-mcgorry-defends-early-intervention-on-youth-mental-health/ (12 December 2020)..

279   Patrick McGorry defends early intervention on youth mental health, Croakey the Crikey Health Blog August 17, 2010. https://www.croakey.org/patrick-mcgorry-defends-early-intervention-on-youth-mental-health/ (12 December 2020)..

280   Patrick McGorry defends early intervention on youth mental health, Croakey the Crikey Health Blog August 17, 2010 https://www.croakey.org/patrick-mcgorry-defends-early-intervention-on-youth-mental-health/ (12 December 2020)..

281   Australian Bureau of Statistics. National Health Survey: First Results, 2017-18 Mental and Behavioural Conditions. 4364.0.55.001, 28 May 2019 https://www.abs.gov.au/ausstats/abs@.nsf/Lookup/by%20Subject/4364.0.55.001~2017-18~Main%20Features~Mental%20and%20behavioural%20conditions~70 (accessed 30 June 2020).

282   Grand View Research, Market Research Report — Attention Deficit Hyperactivity Disorder (ADHD) Market Analysis Report By Drug Type (Stimulant, Non-stimulant), By Demographic, By Distribution Channel (Hospital & Retail Pharmacy), And Segment Forecasts, 2019 – 2025. February 2019. Available at https://www.grandviewresearch.com/industry-analysis/attention-deficit-hyperactivity-disorder-adhd-market (accessed 15 June 2020).

283   American Psychiatric Association (2013), Diagnostic and Statistical Manual of Mental Disorders. Fifth Edition, (DSM5) pp. 59-66.
284   American Psychiatric Association (2013), Diagnostic and Statistical Manual of Mental Disorders. Fifth Edition, (DSM5) pp. 59-66.
285   American Psychiatric Association (2013), Diagnostic and Statistical Manual of Mental Disorders. Fifth Edition, (DSM5) p. 60.
286   American Psychiatric Association (2013), Diagnostic and Statistical Manual of Mental Disorders. Fifth Edition, (DSM5) p. 61.
287   Low Keath, Turning to Adderall for Weight Loss, verywell mind. 8 January 2020.. https://www.verywellmind.com/adderall-rapid-weight-loss-speed-diet-3972108 (accessed 15 June 2020).
288   Table 5. Total number of patients treated with PBS-listed ADHD medicines by age group and gender per calendar year. Attention Deficit Hyperactivity Disorder: Utilisation Analysis Drug utilisation sub-committee (DUSC) May 2018 p19 http://www.pbs.gov.au/industry/listing/participants/public-release-docs/2018-05/adhd-dusc-prd-2018-05-final.pdf (accessed 15 June 2020).
289   American Psychiatric Association, 'DSM-5 Development, Proposed Revision', Attention Deficit/Hyperactivity Disorder. Was available at http://www.dsm5.org/ProposedRevision/Pages/proposedrevision.aspx?rid=383 (accessed 25 July 2011 but is no longer available)..
290   DSM-IV (p87) states 'The clinician should therefore gather information from multiple sources (e.g. parents, teachers) and inquire about the individual's behavior in a variety of situations within each setting. However DSM5 states 'In children and young adolescents, the diagnosis should be based on information obtained from parents and teachers. When direct teacher reports cannot be obtained, weight should be given to information provided to parents by teachers that describe the child's behavior and performance at school'..
291   For example one of the hyperactive/impulsive diagnostic criteria in DSM-IV states; "often leaves seat in classroom or in other situations in which remaining seated is expected". This was replaced in DSM5 with is "often restless during activities when others are seated (may leave his or her place in the classroom, office or other workplace, or in other situations that require remaining seated)"..
292   Department of Health and Ageing, Letter to Martin Whitely MLA dated 21 April 2012..
293   Australian Government Pharmaceutical Benefits Scheme Drug Utilisation Sub-Committee (DUSC) Attention Deficit Hyperactivity Disorder: Utilisation Analysis, Public Release Document, May 2018 DUSC Meeting. Table 5 on page 11. Available at http://www.pbs.gov.au/industry/listing/participants/public-release-docs/2018-05/adhd-dusc-prd-2018-05-final.pdf (accessed 5 January 2019).
294   Department of Health and Ageing, Medicare Australia. Self-generated report from http://medicarestatistics.humanservices.gov.au/statistics/mbs_item.jsp.
295   Other less commonly used brand names for methylphenidate include Methylin, Daytrana, Rubifen, Equasym and Metadate..
296   Kapvay highlights of prescribing information. Available at https://www.accessdata.fda.gov/drugsatfda_docs/label/2010/022331s001s002lbl.pdf (accessed 15 June 2020).
297   Intuniv highlights of prescribing information. Available at https://www.accessdata.fda.gov/drugsatfda_docs/label/2013/022037s009lbl.pdf (accessed 15 June 2020).
298   Rx List Website – Desoxyn https://www.rxlist.com/desoxyn-drug.htm (accessed 15 June 2020).
299   For more detail see PsychWatch Australia website ADHD information page. https://www.psychwatchaustralia.com/treating-adhd (accessed 15 June 2020).
300   Larry S. Goldman, Myron Genel, Rebecca J. Bezman, Priscilla J. Slanetz, for the Council on Scientific Affairs, American Medical Association, 'Diagnosis and treatment of attention-deficit/hyperactivity disorder in children and adolescents', Journal of the American Medical Association, 279(14), pp. 1100–07. https://pubmed.ncbi.nlm.nih.gov/9546570/ (accessed 15 June 2020).
301   Professor Stephen Houghton, Psychologist/University Professor, Graduate School of Education, University of Western Australia, transcript of evidence given to Inquiry into Attention Deficit Disorder and Attention Deficit Hyperactivity Disorder in Western Australia, in Perth on 26 November 2003..
302   Schneider, H., & Eisenberg, D. (2006). Who receives a diagnosis of attention-deficit/hyperactivity disorder in the United States elementary school population? Pediatrics, 117, e601– e609. https://pediatrics.aappublications.org/content/117/4/e601.short?casa_token=g8uS94iSbysAAAAA:RzdL-

CNxf8WNbyZlgzOZcw6AiezZVfxO1iw6dR3AM9ndTC4DdvfUqJzFEVH8AA3NBmCPbF3Z-mOoMdgA (accessed 15 June 2020).

303   Hjern A, Weitoft GR, Lindblad F. Social adversity predicts ADHD-medication in school children--a national cohort study. Acta Paediatr. 2010;99(6):920-4. https://onlinelibrary.wiley.com/doi/10.1111/j.1651-2227.2009.01638.x (accessed 15 June 2020).

304   Russell G, Ford T, Rosenberg R, Kelly S. The association of attention deficit hyperactivity disorder with socioeconomic disadvantage: alternative explanations and evidence. *Journal of Child Psychology Psychiatry*. 2014;55(5):436-45. https://acamh.onlinelibrary.wiley.com/doi/full/10.1111/jcpp.12170 (accessed 15 June 2020).

305   Johnston C, Mash EJ, Miller N, Ninowski JE. Parenting in adults with attention-deficit/hyperactivity disorder (ADHD). Clin Psychol Rev. 2012;32(4):215-28. https://europepmc.org/article/med/22459785 (accessed 15 June 2020).

306   Hjern A, Weitoft GR, Lindblad F. Social adversity predicts ADHD-medication in school children--a national cohort study. Acta Paediatr. 2010;99(6):920-4. https://onlinelibrary.wiley.com/doi/10.1111/j.1651-2227.2009.01638.x (accessed 15 June 2020).

307   Weinstein D, Staffelbach D, Biaggio M. Attention-deficit hyperactivity disorder and posttraumatic stress disorder: differential diagnosis in childhood sexual abuse. Clin Psychol Rev. 2000;20(3):359-78. https://www.sciencedirect.com/science/article/abs/pii/S027273589800107X (accessed 15 June 2020).

308   Thakkar VG. Diagnosing the Wrong Deficit. *New York Times*. 27 April 2013. https://www.nytimes.com/2013/04/28/opinion/sunday/diagnosing-the-wrong-deficit.html (accessed 15 June 2020).

309   Schmitt J, Romanos M. Prenatal and perinatal risk factors for attention-deficit/hyperactivity disorder. Arch Pediatr Adolesc Med. 2012;166(11):1074-5. Prenatal and perinatal risk factors for attention-deficit/hyperactivity disorder. https://pubmed.ncbi.nlm.nih.gov/22200325/#:~:text=CONCLUSIONS%3A%20This%20is%20the%20first,to%2040%20years%20after%20birth. (accessed 15 June 2020).

310   McCann D, Barrett A, Cooper A, Crumpler D, Dalen L, Grimshaw K, et al. Food additives and hyperactive behaviour in 3-year-old and 8/9-year-old children in the community: a randomised, double-blinded, placebo-controlled trial. Lancet. 2007;370(9598):1560-7. https://www.thelancet.com/journals/lancet/article/PIIS0140-6736(07)61306-3/fulltext (accessed 15 June 2020).

311   Byun YH, Ha M, Kwon HJ, Hong YC, Leem JH, Sakong J, et al. Mobile phone use, blood lead levels, and attention deficit hyperactivity symptoms in children: a longitudinal study. PLoS One. 2013;8(3):e59742. https://journals.plos.org/plosone/article?id=10.1371/journal.pone.0059742 (accessed 15 June 2020).

312   Western Australia. Parliament. Legislative Assembly. Attention deficit hyperactivity disorder in Western Australia Perth; 2004. https://www.parliament.wa.gov.au/Parliament/commit.nsf/(Report+Lookup+by+Com+ID)/A8838813E981CEE948257831003E9611/$file/ADD%20final%20report%20pdf%20version.pdf (accessed 15 June 2020).

313   Whitely MP. Attention Deficit Hyperactivity Disorder Policy, Practice and Regulatory Capture in Australia 1992–2012 [PhD]. Perth, WA: Curtin University; 2014. https://espace.curtin.edu.au/bitstream/handle/20.500.11937/1776/225953_Whitely%202014.pdf?sequence=2&isAllowed=y (accessed 15 June 2020).

314   Lydia Furman, (2006) What Is Attention-Deficit Hyperactivity Disorder (ADHD)? *Journal of Child Neurology*. Available at https://www.researchgate.net/publication/7354308_What_Is_Attention-Deficit_Hyperactivity_Disorder_ADHD (accessed 15 June 2020).

315   Peter R. Breggin M.D. (1998), Talking back to Ritalin: What doctors aren't telling you about stimulants for children, Common Courage Press, Monroe, Breggin, p. 20..

316   F. Baughman Jnr. The ADHD Fraud: How Psychiatry Makes "Patients" of Normal Children, Trafford Publishing 2006 p.6.

317   Christopher C Pearson. The diagnostic validity of mental health diagnoses in children. *Medical Journal of Australia*. February 2017. https://www.mja.com.au/journal/2017/206/2/diagnostic-validity-mental-health-diagnoses-children (accessed 16 June 2020).

318   González-Carpio Hernández G1, Serrano Selva JP. (2016) Medication and creativity in

Attention Deficit Hyperactivity Disorder (ADHD). Psicothema. Available at https://www.ncbi.nlm.nih.gov/pubmed/26820419 (accessed 16 June 2020).

319   Gene-Jack Wang, et. al. Long-Term Stimulant Treatment Affects Brain Dopamine Transporter Level in Patients with Attention Deficit Hyperactive Disorder. 15 May 2013 https://www.ncbi.nlm.nih.gov/pmc/articles/PMC3655054/ (accessed 16 June 2020).

320   Shaheen E. Lakhan, Annette Kirchgessner (2012) Prescription stimulants in individuals with and without attention deficit hyperactivity disorder: misuse, cognitive impact, and adverse effects; Brain and Behaviour. Available at https://onlinelibrary.wiley.com/doi/full/10.1002/brb3.78.

321   Lisa L. Weyandt et. al., Prescription Stimulant Medication Misuse: Where Are We and Where Do We Go from Here? Experimental and Clinical Psychopharmacology. October 2016 https://www.researchgate.net/publication/312895023_Prescription_Stimulant_Medication_Misuse_Where_Are_We_and_Where_Do_We_Go_From_Here (accessed 16 June 2020).

322   Whitely M. Speed Up and Sit Still; The controversies of ADHD diagnosis and treatment, UWA Publishing 2010 page 39 https://e46126be-5e83-4973-a0fe-598613447990.filesusr.com/ugd/02a3d9_ed087b00ef6d472fb8e2ccf2b9fa3a75.pdf (accessed 16 June 2020).

323   Janet Currie, Mark Stabile, and Lauren Jones. Do Stimulant Medications Improve Educational and Behavioral Outcomes for Children with ADHD? https://www.ncbi.nlm.nih.gov/pmc/articles/PMC4815037/ (accessed 16 June 2020).

324   Janet Currie, Mark Stabile, and Lauren Jones. Do Stimulant Medications Improve Educational and Behavioral Outcomes for Children with ADHD? https://www.ncbi.nlm.nih.gov/pmc/articles/PMC4815037/ (accessed 16 June 2020).

325   Government of Western Australia, Department of Health, Raine ADHD Study: Long-term outcomes associated with stimulant medication in the treatment of ADHD in children, Department of Health, Perth, 2010. http://www.health.wa.gov.au/publications/documents/MICADHD_Raine_ADHD_study_report_022010.pdf (accessed 16 June 2020).

326   Government of Western Australia, Department of Health, Raine ADHD Study: Long-term outcomes associated with stimulant medication in the treatment of ADHD in children, Department of Health, Perth, 2010. http://www.health.wa.gov.au/publications/documents/MICADHD_Raine_ADHD_study_report_022010.pdf (accessed 16 June 2020).

327   Peter Breggin, 'A Critical Analysis of the NIMH Multimodal Treatment Study for Attention-Deficit/Hyperactivity Disorder (The MTA Study)' in *Psychiatric Drug Facts* 2000. Previously available at https://www.researchgate.net/publication/267683330_A_critical_analysis_of_the_NIMH_Multimodal_Treatment_Study_for_Attention-DeficitHyperactivity_Disorder_the_MTA_study (accessed 16 June 2020).

328   The MTA Study was 'the first multisite, cooperative agreement treatment study of children, and the largest psychiatric/psychological treatment trial ever conducted by the (U.S.) National Institute of Mental Health. It examines the effectiveness of Medication vs. Psychosocial treatment vs. their combination for treatment of ADHD and compares these experimental arms to each other and to routine community care.' K. C. Wells, W. E. Pelham, et al., 'Psychosocial treatment strategies in the MTA study: rationale, methods, and critical issues in design and implementation', (abstract), *Journal of Abnormal Child Psychology*, Vol. 28, No. 6, 2000. https://pubmed.ncbi.nlm.nih.gov/11104313/ (accessed 16 June 2020).

329   The study was sponsored by the National Institute of Mental Health (NIMH) and conducted at six separate US sites. At each site, the study compared four treatment conditions: medication management alone, combined medication management and behavioural therapy, behavioural therapy, and community care. The average age of the children was eight and 80 per cent were boys. For more information, see The MTA Cooperative Group, 'A 14-Month Randomized Clinical Trial of Treatment Strategies for Attention-Deficit/Hyperactivity Disorder', *Archives of General Psychiatry*, 56, 1999, p. 1073. https://jamanetwork.com/journals/jamapsychiatry/fullarticle/205525 (accessed 16 June 2020).

330   Merle G. Paule, Andrew S. Rowland, Sherry A. Ferguson, et al., 'Attention deficit/hyperactivity disorder: characteristics, interventions, and models' in *Neurotoxicology and Teratology*, Vol. 22, No. 5, 2000, p. 631. https://www.sciencedirect.com/science/article/abs/pii/S0892036200000957 (accessed 16 June 2020).

331   Allegra Stratton, 'Questions raised about drugs as treatment for ADHD sufferers', *The Guardian*, 12 November 2007.

332   Brooke Molina, Kate Flory, Stephen P. Hinshaw et al., 'Delinquent Behavior and Emerging Substance Use in the MTA at 36 Months: Prevalence, Course, and Treatment Effects', *Journal of the American Academy of Child & Adolescent Psychiatry,* Vol. 46 No. 8, August 2007: pp. 1028–1040; https://www.sciencedirect.com/science/article/abs/pii/S0890856709615537 (accessed 16 June 2020).
333   Allegra Stratton, 'Questions raised about drugs as treatment for ADHD sufferers', *The Guardian,* November 12th, 2007.
334   Swanson J.M. et al. Young adult outcomes in the follow-up of the multimodal treatment study of attention-deficit/hyperactivity disorder: symptom persistence, source discrepancy, and height suppression. *Journal of Child Psychiatry and Psychology.* 2017. https://onlinelibrary.wiley.com/doi/abs/10.1111/jcpp.12684?fbclid=IwAR3_uAkzB7jKfx-qdOXYMIhPi1IyeAZ_h7_JRyv-PTLjqREdxqAG92RykaU (Accessed 17 May 2020).
335   Joseph M. Rey, 'In the long run, skills are as good as pills for attention deficit hyperactivity disorder', *The Medical Journal of Australia,* 188:3, 2008, p. 134. https://www.mja.com.au/journal/2008/188/3/long-run-skills-are-good-pills-attention-deficit-hyperactivity-disorder (accessed 16 June 2020).
336   Whitely M, Raven M, Timimi S, Jureidini J, Phillimore J, Leo J, Moncrieff J, Landman P, Attention deficit hyperactivity disorder late birthdate effect common in both high and low prescribing international jurisdictions: systematic review, *Journal of Child Psychology and Psychiatry,* October 2018. https://onlinelibrary.wiley.com/doi/abs/10.1111/jcpp.12991 (accessed 16 June 2020).
337   Whitely M, Lester L, Phillimore J, Robinson S, Influence of birth month of Western Australian children on the probability of being treated for ADHD, *Medical Journal of Australia,* 2017. https://www.mja.com.au/journal/2017/206/2/influence-birth-month-probability-western-australian-children-being-treated-adhd (accessed 16 June 2020).
338   Timothy J. Layton et. al. Attention Deficit–Hyperactivity Disorder and Month of School Enrolment. New England Journal of Medicine November 2018 https://www.researchgate.net/publication/329264480_Attention_Deficit-Hyperactivity_Disorder_and_Month_of_School_Enrollment (accessed 16 June 2020).
339   Gordon S. Youngest in Class Diagnosed More Often With ADHD. WebMd, 23 September 2019 https://www.webmd.com/add-adhd/news/20190923/youngest-in-class-diagnosed-more-often-with-adhd#1 (accessed 16 June 2020).
340   Evans, W.N., Morrill, M.S., & Parente, S.T. (2010). Measuring inappropriate medical diagnosis and treatment in survey data: The case of ADHD among school-age children. *Journal of Health Economics,* 29, 657– 673. https://www.sciencedirect.com/science/article/abs/pii/S0167629610000962 (accessed 16 June 2020).
341   Morrow, R.L., Garland, E.J., Wright, J.M., Maclure, M., Taylor, S., & Dormuth, C.R. (2012). Influence of relative age on diagnosis and treatment of attention-deficit/hyperactivity disorder in children. CMAJ, 184, 755– 762. https://www.ncbi.nlm.nih.gov/pmc/articles/PMC3328520/ (accessed 16 June 2020).
342   Zoega, H., Valdimarsdottir, U.A., & Hernandez-Diaz, S. (2012). Age, academic performance, and stimulant prescribing for ADHD: A nationwide cohort study. Pediatrics, 130, 1012– 1018. https://www.ncbi.nlm.nih.gov/pmc/articles/PMC3507253/ (accessed 16 June 2020).
343   Frances, A. (2016/2017, 23 May/24 May) Conclusive Proof ADHD Is Overdiagnosed. *Huffington Post.* https://www.huffpost.com/entry/conclusive-proof-adhd-is-overdiagnosed_b_10107214 (accessed 16 June 2020).
344   Frances, A. (2015). Don't throw out the baby with the bath water. *Australian and New Zealand Journal of Psychiatry,* 49, 577. https://journals.sagepub.com/doi/10.1177/0004867415579467 (accessed 16 June 2020).
345   Halldner, L., Tillander, A., Lundholm, C., Boman, M., Langstrom, N., Larsson, H., & Lichtenstein, P. (2014). Relative immaturity and ADHD: Findings from nationwide registers, parent- and self-reports. *Journal of Child Psychology and Psychiatry,* 55, 897– 904. https://acamh.onlinelibrary.wiley.com/doi/abs/10.1111/jcpp.12229?identityKey=4c3b91fb-9215-4f20-ad10-d275eb047556&regionCode=ES&wol1URL=%2Fdoi%2F10.1111%2Fjcpp.12229%2Fabstract (accessed 16 June 2020).
346   Sayal, K., Chudal, R., Hinkka-Yli-Salomaki, S., Joelsson, P., & Sourander, A. (2017). Relative

age within the school year and diagnosis of attention-deficit hyperactivity disorder: A nationwide population-based study. Lancet Psychiatry, 4, 868– 875. https://nottingham-repository.worktribe.com/output/887026/relative-age-within-the-school-year-and-diagnosis-of-attention-deficit-hyperactivity-disorder-a-nationwide-population-based-study (accessed 16 June 2020).

347   Chen, M.H., Lan, W.H., Bai, Y.M., Huang, K.L., Su, T.P., Tsai, S.J., & Hsu, J.W. (2016). Influence of relative age on diagnosis and treatment of attention-deficit hyperactivity disorder in Taiwanese children. *Journal of Pediatrics*, 172, 162– 167. e1. https://www.jpeds.com/article/S0022-3476(16)00160-8/abstract (accessed 16 June 2020).

348   Whitely, M., Lester, L., Phillimore, J., & Robinson, S. (2017). Influence of birth month on the probability of Western Australian children being treated for ADHD. *Medical Journal of Australia*, 206, 85. https://www.mja.com.au/journal/2017/206/2/influence-birth-month-probability-western-australian-children-being-treated-adhd (accessed 16 June 2020).

349   Librero, J., Izquierdo-Maria, R., Garcia-Gil, M., & Peiro, S. (2015). Children's relative age in class and medication for attention-deficit/hyperactivity disorder. A population-based study in a health department in Spain. Medicina Clínica (Barc), 145, 471– 476. https://www.researchgate.net/publication/301779731_Children's_relative_age_in_class_and_medication_for_attention-deficithyperactivity_disorder_A_population-based_study_in_a_health_department_in_Spain (accessed 16 June 2020).

350   Allen Frances, Don't throw out the baby with the bath water, *Australian and New Zealand Journal of Psychiatry*, April 28, 2015 https://journals.sagepub.com/doi/full/10.1177/0004867415579467 (accessed 16 June 2020).

351   Curtin University website 2017 Research and Engagement Award winners. https://news.curtin.edu.au/stories/2017-research-engagement-award-winners/ (accessed 16 June 2020).

352   See https://wiley.altmetric.com/details/49661341#score (accessed 16 June 2020).

353   Kate Sikora, We're turning our children psychotic with ADHD medication, *The Daily Telegraph* October 13, 2009. https://www.dailytelegraph.com.au/archive/z-resources/were-turning-our-children-psychotic/news-story/ec79dc808c9e972a2e276d77bdb49a33 (accessed 16 June 2020).

354   'Medicating our children', Reportage Online: *Magazine of the Australian Centre for Independent Journalism*, 22 December 2009. Was previously available at http://www.reportageonline.com/2009/12/medicating-our-children/ (accessed 29 June 2011).

355   Peter R. Breggin M.D. (1998), Talking back to Ritalin: *What doctors aren't telling you about stimulants for children*, Common Courage Press, Monroe, Breggin, p. 236..

356   Paul H. Wender, *Attention-Deficit Hyperactivity Disorder in Adults,* Oxford University Press, New York, 1995, p. 20.

357   Paul H. Wender, *Attention-Deficit Hyperactivity Disorder in Adults,* Oxford University Press, New York, 1995, pp. 139–49.

358   Marian S. McDonagh, Kim Petersen, et al., *Drug Class Review on Pharmacologic Treatments for ADHD: Final Report Update 2,* Portland, Oregon Health & Science University (2007). Available at https://www.ohsu.edu/sites/default/files/2019-01/ADHD_final-report_update-2_NOV_07.pdf (accessed 17 June 2020)..

359   Alexander Otto, 'Are ADHD drugs safe? Report finds little proof', *The News Tribune*, 13 September 2005. Previously available at http://www.playattention.com/attention-deficit/articles/are-adhd-drugs-safe-report-finds-little-proof (accessed 12 May 2007)..

360   Marian S. McDonagh, Kim Petersen, et al., *Drug Class Review on Pharmacologic Treatments for ADHD: Final Report Update 2,* Portland, Oregon Health & Science University (2007). Available at https://www.ohsu.edu/sites/default/files/2019-01/ADHD_final-report_update-2_NOV_07.pdf (accessed 17 June 2020).

361   Marian S. McDonagh, Kim Petersen, et al., *Drug Class Review on Pharmacologic Treatments for ADHD: Final Report Update 2,* Portland, Oregon Health & Science University (2007). Available at https://www.ohsu.edu/sites/default/files/2019-01/ADHD_final-report_update-2_NOV_07.pdf (accessed 17 June 2020).

362   Marian S. McDonagh, Kim Petersen, et al., *Drug Class Review on Pharmacologic Treatments for ADHD: Final Report Update 2,* Portland, Oregon Health & Science University 2007. p 24 Available at https://www.ohsu.edu/sites/default/files/2019-01/ADHD_final-report_update-2_NOV_07.pdf (accessed 17 June 2020).

363   Marian S. McDonagh, Kim Petersen, et al., *Drug Class Review on Pharmacologic Treatments for ADHD: Final Report Update 2,* Portland, Oregon Health & Science University 2007 p 20. Available at https://www.ohsu.edu/sites/default/files/2019-01/ADHD_final-report_update-2_NOV_07.pdf (accessed 17 June 2020).

364   Marian S. McDonagh, Kim Petersen, et al., *Drug Class Review on Pharmacologic Treatments for ADHD: Final Report Update 2,* Portland, Oregon Health & Science University 2007 p 16. Available at https://www.ohsu.edu/sites/default/files/2019-01/ADHD_final-report_update-2_NOV_07.pdf (accessed 17 June 2020).

365   Marian S. McDonagh, Kim Petersen, et al., *Drug Class Review on Pharmacologic Treatments for ADHD: Final Report Update 2,* Portland, Oregon Health & Science University 2007 p.21. Available at https://www.ohsu.edu/sites/default/files/2019-01/ADHD_final-report_update-2_NOV_07.pdf (accessed 17 June 2020).

366   Alexander Otto, 'Are ADHD drugs safe? Report finds little proof', *The News Tribune,* 13 September 2005. Previously available at http://www.playattention.com/attention-deficit/articles/are-adhd-drugs-safe-report-finds-little-proof (accessed 12 May 2007)..

367   Alan Schwarz, ADHD Nation: The disorder. The drugs. The inside story. Little Brown, 2016. .

368   Sami Timimi, et al., 'A Critique of the International Consensus Statement on ADHD', *Clinical Child and Family Psychology Review,* Vol. 7, No. 1, 2004, p. 59. https://www.researchgate.net/publication/8585093_A_Critique_of_the_International_Consensus_Statement_on_ADHD (accessed 17 June 2020).

369   Sami Timimi, et al., 'A Critique of the International Consensus Statement on ADHD', *Clinical Child and Family Psychology Review,* Vol. 7, No. 1, 2004, p. 59. https://www.researchgate.net/publication/8585093_A_Critique_of_the_International_Consensus_Statement_on_ADHD (accessed 17 June 2020).

370   Sami Timimi, et al., 'A Critique of the International Consensus Statement on ADHD', *Clinical Child and Family Psychology Review,* Vol. 7, No. 1, 2004, p. 60. https://www.researchgate.net/publication/8585093_A_Critique_of_the_International_Consensus_Statement_on_ADHD (accessed 17 June 2020).

371   Peter R. Breggin, M.D., *Talking Back to Ritalin: What Doctors Aren't Telling You about Stimulants for Children,* Common Courage Press, Monroe, 1998, p. 358..

372   Kelland, K. Study finds first evidence that ADHD is genetic, Reuters, 30 September 2010. http://www.reuters.com/article/2010/09/30/us-adhd-genes-idUSTRE68S5UD20100930 (accessed 22 November 2012).

373   Landau, E. (2010) ADHD is a genetic condition, study says, CNN Health, 29 September 2010. Available at http://thechart.blogs.cnn.com/2010/09/29/adhd-is-a-genetic-condition-study-says/ (accessed 14 November 2012).

374   *ABC Online News* Study finds genetic link to ADHD, 30 September 2010. Available at http://www.abc.net.au/news/2010-09-30/study-finds-genetic-link-to-adhd/2280292 (accessed 22 November 2012).

375   *ABC Online News* Study finds genetic link to ADHD, 30 September 2010. Available at http://www.abc.net.au/news/2010-09-30/study-finds-genetic-link-to-adhd/2280292 (accessed 22 November 2012) .

376   Williams, N.M., Zaharieva, I., Martin, A., Langley, K., et al (2010) Rare chromosomal deletions and duplications in attention-deficit hyperactivity disorder: a genome-wide analysis, *The Lancet,* 376, 1401-1408 https://www.thelancet.com/journals/lancet/article/PIIS0140-6736(10)61109-9/fulltext (accessed 17 June 2020).

377   Williams, N.M., Zaharieva, I., Martin, A., Langley, K., et al (2010) Rare chromosomal deletions and duplications in attention-deficit hyperactivity disorder: a genome-wide analysis, *The Lancet,* 376, 1401-1408 https://www.thelancet.com/journals/lancet/article/PIIS0140-6736(10)61109-9/fulltext (accessed 17 June 2020).

378   Williams, N.M., Thapar, A. et al (2011) Structural variations in attention-deficit hyperactivity disorder — Authors' reply, *The Lancet,* 377, 378. https://www.thelancet.com/journals/lancet/article/PIIS0140-6736(11)60121-9/fulltext (accessed 17 June 2020).

379   Chapter 2 of Retz W, Klein RG (eds): Attention-Deficit Hyperactivity Disorder (ADHD) in Adults. Key Issues in Mental Health. Basel, Karger, 2010, vol 176, pp 38–57 Family and Twin Studies in Attention-Deficit Hyperactivity Disorder Christine Margarete Freitaga Wolfgang Retzb https://

www.researchgate.net/publication/281941504_Family_and_Twin_Studies_in_Attention-Deficit_
Hyperactivity_Disorder (accessed 17 June 2020).

380   Larsson, H., Chang, Z., D'Onofrio, B. M., & Lichtenstein, P. (2013). The heritability of clinically
diagnosed attention deficit hyperactivity disorder across the lifespan. *Psychological Medicine*, 44(10),
2223–2229. https://www.ncbi.nlm.nih.gov/pubmed/24107258 (accessed 17 June 2020).

381   Bob Jacobs, Youth Affairs Network of Queensland, Being an Educated Consumer of 'ADHD'
Research, Youth Affairs Network of Queensland, 2005 http://www.atca.com.au/wp-content/
uploads/2012/09/Bob-Jacobs-being-an-educated-consumer-of-ADHD-research.pdf (accessed 17
June 2020).

382   Neelima Choahan. Australians with ADHD may be missing out on diagnosis and treatment,
News GP 18 Sep 2018 https://www1.racgp.org.au/newsgp/clinical/australians-with-adhd-might-be-
missing-out-on-prop.

383   GlaxoSmithKline, *Prescribing Information – Dexedrine (dextroamphetamine sulphate)*. FDA
https://www.accessdata.fda.gov/drugsatfda_docs/label/2007/017078s042lbl.pdf (accessed 17 June 2020).

384   American Psychiatric Association, *Treatments of Psychiatric Disorders: a task force report of the
American Psychiatric Association,* 1st ed., 1989.

385   American Psychiatric Association, Diagnostic and Statistical Manual of Mental Disorders. Fifth
Edition, 2013 p. 563.

386   Parliament of Western Australia, *Hansard,* Martin Whitely MLA, Thursday, 25 February 2010,
pp. 259b–293a..

387   Whitely MP. Attention Deficit Hyperactivity Disorder Policy, Practice and Regulatory Capture
in Australia 1992–2012 [PhD]. Perth, WA: Curtin University; 2014. https://espace.curtin.edu.au/
bitstream/handle/20.500.11937/1776/225953_Whitely%202014.pdf?sequence=2&isAllowed=y
(accessed 17 June 2020).

388   Whitely MP. Attention Deficit Hyperactivity Disorder Policy, Practice and Regulatory Capture
in Australia 1992–2012 [PhD]. Perth, WA: Curtin University; 2014. https://espace.curtin.edu.au/
bitstream/handle/20.500.11937/1776/225953_Whitely%202014.pdf?sequence=2&isAllowed=y
(accessed 15 June 2020).

389   Whitely MP. Attention Deficit Hyperactivity Disorder Policy, Practice and Regulatory Capture
in Australia 1992–2012 [PhD]. Perth, WA: Curtin University; 2014. https://espace.curtin.edu.au/
bitstream/handle/20.500.11937/1776/225953_Whitely%202014.pdf?sequence=2&isAllowed=y
(accessed 15 June 2020).

390   Whitely M. ADHD debate clouded by preconceptions and undisclosed conflicts of interest.
Australian & New Zealand Journal of Psychiatry. 2013;47(10):956-8. https://journals.sagepub.com/
doi/abs/10.1177/0004867413498270 (accessed 15 June 2020).

391   Department of Health Western Australia. Western Australian Stimulant Regulatory Scheme
2017 Annual Report. Pharmaceutical Services Branch, Health Protection Group; 2017. https://ww2.
health.wa.gov.au/~/media/Files/Corporate/general%20documents/medicines%20and%20poisons/
PDF/Stimulant-Regulatory-Scheme-2017-Annual-Report.pdf (accessed 17 June 2020).

392   Whitely M. Allsop S. Look west for Australian evidence of the relationship between
amphetamine-type stimulant prescribing and meth/amphetamine use. Drug and Alcohol Review
April 2020 https://onlinelibrary.wiley.com/doi/full/10.1111/dar.13067 (accessed 17 June 2020).

393   Drug and Alcohol Office WA. Australian Secondary School Alcohol and Drug (ASSAD) Report
2005. Mt Lawley WA 2007.

394   Government of Western Australia Mental Health Commission. Illicit Drug Trends in Western
Australia: Australian School Students Alcohol and Drug Survey 2017. 15 January 2019..

395   Government of Western Australia Department of Health, Western Australian Stimulant
Regulatory Scheme 2017 Annual Report. 2019 https://ww2.health.wa.gov.au/~/media/Files/
Corporate/general%20documents/medicines%20and%20poisons/PDF/Stimulant-Regulatory-
Scheme-2017-Annual-Report.pdf (accessed 17 June 2020).

396   Whitely MP. Attention Deficit Hyperactivity Disorder Policy, Practice and Regulatory Capture
in Australia 1992–2012 [PhD]. Perth, WA: Curtin University; 2014. https://espace.curtin.edu.au/
bitstream/handle/20.500.11937/1776/225953_Whitely%202014.pdf?sequence=2&isAllowed=y
(accessed 15 June 2020).

397   Whitely M. Allsop S. Look west for Australian evidence of the relationship between amphetamine-type stimulant prescribing and meth/amphetamine use. *Drug and Alcohol Review* April 2020 https://onlinelibrary.wiley.com/doi/full/10.1111/dar.13067 (accessed 17 June 2020).

398   Owens B. Harvard scientists disciplined for not declaring ties to drug companies, Nature.com 4 July 2011. http://blogs.nature.com/news/2011/07/harvard_scientists_disciplined.html (accessed 20 June 2020).

399   People Professor Ian Hickie. University of Sydney website https://www.sydney.edu.au/medicine-health/about/our-people/academic-staff/ian-hickie.html (accessed 19 June 2020).

400   Publications for Ian Hickie. Available at https://www.sydney.edu.au/medicine-health/about/our-people/academic-staff/ian-hickie.html (accessed 19 June 2020).

401   Government of Western Australia, Department of Health, Raine ADHD Study: Long-term outcomes associated with stimulant medication in the treatment of ADHD in children, Department of Health, Perth, 2010. https://ww2.health.wa.gov.au/-/media/Files/Corporate/Reports-and-publications/PDF/MICADHD_Raine_ADHD_Study_report_022010.pdf (accessed 10 December 2020).

402   Interview with Professor Ian Hickie on ABC PM program with Mark Colvin, 'New Research Reignites Debate over ADHD', 17 February 2010. Available at http://www.abc.net.au/pm/content/2010/s2822748.htm (accessed 19 July 2020).

403   Hickie I. (2018). Curriculum Vitae: Ian Hickie AM MD FRANZCP FASSA. Available at: http://api.profiles.sydney.edu.au/AcademicProfiles/profile/resource?urlid=ian.hickie&type=cv (Accessed 18 November 2019).

404   Hickie I. (2004). Can we reduce the burden of depression? The Australian experience with beyondblue: the national depression initiative. *Australasian Psychiatry*, 12(suppl. 1), S38-S46. https://journals.sagepub.com/doi/10.1080/j.1039-8562.2004.02097.x-2 (accessed 10 December 2020)..

405   Hickie, Ian B. (2004). Reducing the burden of depression: are we making progress in Australia? *MJA, 181*(7), S4-S5. http://www.mja.com.au/public/issues/181_07_041004/hic10389_fm.html. (accessed 2 August 2020).

406   beyondblue the national depression initiative 2001 Annual Report p.18 https://resources.beyondblue.org.au/prism/ile?token=BL/0001 (accessed 19 July 2020).

407   Wooldridge, Michael. (2000). Wooldridge appoints Kennett to tackle one of Australia's leading causes of lost days (media release) 14 March 2000. Canberra: Australian Government Department of Health and Ageing. http://www.health.gov.au/internet/main/publishing.nsf/Content/health-mediarel-yr2000-mw-mw20024.htm (accessed 4 March 2011).

408   Wooldridge was Minister for Health and Family Services 1996-1998, then continued as Minister for Health and Aged Care 1998-2001.

409   Beyond Blue Limited Annual Financial Statements 2018/19 https://www.beyondblue.org.au/docs/default-source/default-document-library/beyond-blue-annual-highlights-2018-19-web.pdf. (accessed 19 July 2020).

410   Hickie, I. (2004). Reducing the burden of depression: are we making progress in Australia? MJA, 181(7), S4-S5. https://www.mja.com.au/journal/2004/181/7/reducing-burden-depression-are-we-making-progress-australia (accessed 2 August 2020).

411   http://www.smh.com.au/articles/2004/06/25/1088144980637.html.

412   Robotham, Julie. (2004, June 26). It's professors at 10 paces as drugs row gets personal. *Sydney Morning Herald*. http://www.smh.com.au/articles/2004/06/25/1088144980637.html (accessed 10 January 2020).

413   Hickie, Ian B., Davenport, Tracey A., Naismith, Sharon L., & Scott, Elizabeth M., on behalf of the SPHERE National Secretariat. (2001). SPHERE: A National Depression Project. *Medical Journal of Australia*, 175 (Suppl.) S4-S5.

414   Parker, Gordon B. (2000). Depressed Australians: Should we worry? *MJA, 173*(9), 452-453. www.mja.com.au/public/issues/173_09_061100/parker/parker.html (accessed 22 July 2020).

415   University of New South Wales (2002) UNSW Professor to Head Major Mental Health Initiative. https://web.archive.org/web/20040928100205/http:/www.unsw.edu.au/news/adv/articles/2002/feb/ProfessorToHeadMajor.html (accessed 31 July 2020).

416   Hickie I. (2018). Curriculum Vitae: Ian Hickie AM MD FRANZCP FASSA. Available at: http://api.profiles.sydney.edu.au/AcademicProfiles/profile/resource?urlid=ian.hickie&type=cv (Accessed 18 November 2019).

417   Hickie I, Hadzi-Pavlovic D, Scott E, Davenport T, Koschera A, & Naismith S. (1998). SPHERE: A national depression project. *Australasian Psychiatry*, 6(5), 248-250. https://journals.sagepub.com/doi/10.3109/10398569809084854 (accessed 10 December 2020). (p. 249).

418   Scott, E. (2008) BMRI Doctor Elizabeth Margaret Scott [CV]. http://web.archive.org/web/20080723223118/http://www.bmri.org.au/scott.html (16 August 2020).

419   Hickie, Ian B., Davenport, Tracey A., Naismith, Sharon L., & Scott, Elizabeth M., on behalf of the SPHERE National Secretariat. (2001). Conclusions about the assessment and management of common mental disorders in Australian general practice SPHERE: A National Depression Project. *Medical Journal of Australia*, 175(Suppl.), S52-S55. (p. S54).

420   Lamont, L. (2001, February 1). Depression more common than asthma: GPs. *Sydney Morning Herald*. https://www.newspapers.com/newspage/121428219/ (accessed 10 December 2020)..

421   Sweet M. A tall fellow who talks a lot. *Australian Doctor*. 2001 http://www.sweetcommunication.com.au/files/ausdoc/profiles/2001/hickie.pdf (accessed 5 December 2020)..

422   Baker, Richard. (2006, August 8). Mental health takes industry pills. *The Age*. http://www.theage.com.au/news/national/mental-health-takes-industry-pills/2006/08/07/1154802820416.html (accessed 22 July 2020).

423   Lifeblood website. Medical Education. 29 March 2010 https://web.archive.org/web/20100329155407/http://lifeblood.com.au/cs_1.html (accessed 31 July 2020).

424   Davies, Julie-Anne. GP jaunts 'boosted' drug sales. *The Australian*. 10 July 2010. https://www.theaustralian.com.au/news/health-science/gp-jaunts-boosted-drug-sales/news-story/37e3522ccf14533c143f32424d6109aa (accessed 10 December 2020).

425   Scott E. (2008) CV. Brain and Mind Institute website 23 July 2008 http://web.archive.org/web/20080723223118/http://www.bmri.org.au/scott.html (accessed 10 December 2020)..

426   Australian Securities & Investments Commission (12 January 2011). Company extract: Devine Publishing Pty Ltd. eSearch Pty Ltd.

427   Australian Securities & Investments Commission (4 March 2011). Business Names Extract – New South Wales: Educational Health Solutions..

428   Australian Securities & Investments Commission (12 January 2011). Company extract: Strange & Duncan Pty Ltd.

429   Lifeblood (2007) Networks. https://web.archive.org/web/20071228102737/http://www.lifeblood.com.au/networks.html (13 December 2020).

430   Beyondblue. SPHERE: A National Depression Project. *Medical Journal of Australia*, 175(Suppl.) 16 July 2001. https://onlinelibrary.wiley.com/toc/13265377/2001/175/S1 (accessed 10 December 2020)..

431   Phillips, N., Oldmeadow, M. J., & Krapivansky, N. (2002, February 18). SPHERE: A National Depression Project. *Medical Journal of Australia*, 176(4), 193-194. https://onlinelibrary.wiley.com/doi/full/10.5694/j.1326-5377.2002.tb04364.x (5 December 2020).

432   Clarke, David M., & McKenzie, Dean P. (2003, April). An examination of the efficiency of the 12-item SPHERE questionnaire as a screening instrument for common mental disorders in primary care. *Australian and New Zealand Journal of Psychiatry*, 37(2), 236-239.

433   Hickie IB, Davenport TA, Hadzi-Pavlovic D, et al. (2001). Development of a simple screening tool for common mental disorders in general practice. *Medical Journal of Australia*, 175(2 Suppl): S10-S17.

434   Spitzer, Robert L., Williams, Janet B. W., Kroenke, Kurt, Linzer, Mark, deGruy, Frank V. 3rd, Hahn, Steven R., Brody, David, & Johnson, Jeffrey G. (1994). Utility of a New Procedure for Diagnosing Mental Disorders in Primary Care: The PRIME-MD 1000 Study. *JAMA, 272*(22), 1749-1756. https://jamanetwork.com/journals/jama/fullarticle/383992 (16 August 2020).

435   Hickie IB, Davenport TA, Scott EM, Hadzi-Pavlovic D, Naismith SL, Koschera A. (2001). Unmet need for recognition of common mental disorders in Australian general practice. *Medical Journal of Australia*, 175(2 Suppl.), S18-24. (p. S19, box 1).

436   Hickie, Ian B., Davenport, Tracey A., Naismith, Sharon L., & Scott, Elizabeth M., on behalf of the SPHERE National Secretariat. (2001). Conclusions about the assessment and management of common mental disorders in Australian general practice SPHERE: A National Depression Project. *Medical Journal of Australia*, 175(Suppl.), S52-S55. (p. S52).

437   Beyondblue. (2001) The SPHERE Project: key findings. GP Review, 5(8), 11.

438   Milligan, Louise. (2001, 14-15 July). 60pc of GPs' patients mentally ill. *The Weekend Australian*, p. 3.

439   Robotham, Julie. (2001, July 16). Six in 10 GP patients have mental illness: study. *Sydney Morning Herald.*

440   Raven, M. (2012). Depression and antidepressants in Australia and beyond: A critical public health analysis. [dissertation/PhD thesis (Chapter 9 pp. 379-424). University of Wollongong. http:// ro.uow.edu.au/theses/3686/ (accessed July 2020).

441   Yahoo7 (2011, June 22). 7News exposes medical scandal. Yahoo! News. https://au.news.yahoo. com/7news-exposes-medical-scandal-9690341.html (accessed 10 December 2020)..

442   Burrows, Graham D. Editorial. *Depression Awareness Journal,* 5, 7 and 9, inside front cover. July 1998, February 1999 and August 1999.

443   Hickie, I., Scott, E., Davenport, T., Gillies, K., Ricci, C. (2003). 'SPHERE: a national depression project'. Providing enhanced care in the general practice setting. *Depression Awareness Journal,* 12, 6-7.

444   Givney, J. Depression & sleep disturbance: A case history. *Depression Awareness Journal,* August 1999 p.8.

445   Givney, J. Depression & sleep disturbance: A case history. *Depression Awareness Journal,* August 1999 p.8.

446   Hickie I, Hadzi-Pavlovic D, Scott E, Davenport T, Koschera A, Naismith S. (1998). SPHERE: A national depression project. *Australasian Psychiatry,* 6(5), 248-250.

447   Hickie, IB., Davenport, TA., Scott, EM., Hadzi-Pavlovic, D, Naismith, S L., & Koschera, A (2001). Unmet need for recognition of common mental disorders in Australian general practice. *Medical Journal of Australia,* 175(Suppl.), S18-S24. (p. S23).

448   Beyondblue. SPHERE: A National Depression Project. *Medical Journal of Australia,* 175(Suppl.). 16 July 2001.

449   Australian Government. Department of Health and Ageing 2000-01 Annual Report excerpt available at https://web.archive.org/web/20020225054037/http://www.health.gov.au/pubs/annrep/ ar2001/part2/02_0083.htm (accessed 20 July 2020).

450   Beyond Blue. beyondblue BULLETIN. November 2011. http://pandora.nla.gov.au/ pan/25494/20020711-0000/www.beyondblue.org.au/site/resourcelibrary/beyondblue%20bulletin%20 2001.pdf (accessed 3 August 2020).

451   Baker, Richard. (2006, August 8). Mental health takes industry pills. *The Age.* http://www. theage.com.au/news/national/mental-health-takes-industry-pills/2006/08/07/1154802820416.html (accessed 22 July 2020).

452   beyondblue (2013) SPHERE Questionnaire https://web.archive.org/web/20130209030620/ http://www.beyondblue.org.au/index.aspx?link_id=89.677 (accessed 15 August 2020).

453   Lifeblood (2007). Medical Education. https://web.archive.org/web/20071228102717/http:// www.lifeblood.com.au/cs_1.html (accessed 13 December 2020).

454   Lifeblood website. Medical Education. 29 March 2010 https://web.archive.org/ web/20100329155407/http://lifeblood.com.au/cs_1.html (accessed 31 July 2020).

455   Australian Securities & Investments Commission (2011, March 4) Business Names Extract – New South Wales: Educational Health Solutions.

456   Williams D. Antidepressant drugs ranked in study. Australian Doctor. 4 February 2009 http:// www.australiandoctor.com.au/news/33/0c05ce33.asp (accessed 4 September 2011).

457   Lifeblood website. Philosophy. 29 March 2010 https://web.archive.org/web/20100329160007/ http://lifeblood.com.au/philosophy.html (accessed 3 August 2020).

458   Davies, Julie-Anne. GP jaunts 'boosted' drug sales. *The Australian.* 10 July 2010. https://www. theaustralian.com.au/news/health-science/gp-jaunts-boosted-drug-sales/news-story/37e3522ccf1453 3c143f32424d6109aa (accessed 10 December 2020).

459   Hickie, I. Curriculum vitae: Ian Hickie. Sydney: Brain & Mind Research Institute. 23 August 2009. Sydney: Brain & Mind Research Institute. https://web.archive.org/web/20100331230312/http:// www.bmri.org.au/about/Hickie_CV.pdf (accessed 3 December 2020).

460   Lifeblood. (2010). About SPHERE. https://web.archive.org/web/20100619110405/http://www. spheregp.com.au/about-sphere.aspx (accessed 11 December 2020).

461   Davies, Julie-Anne. GP jaunts 'boosted' drug sales. *The Australian.* 10 July 2010. https://www. theaustralian.com.au/news/health-science/gp-jaunts-boosted-drug-sales/news-story/37e3522ccf1453 3c143f32424d6109aa (accessed 10 December 2020).

462   Davies, Julie-Anne. GP jaunts 'boosted' drug sales. *The Australian.* 10 July 2010. https://www.

theaustralian.com.au/news/health-science/gp-jaunts-boosted-drug-sales/news-story/37e3522ccf1453 3c143f32424d6109aa (accessed 10 December 2020).

463   Hall W. Mant A. Mitchell P. Rendle V. Hickie I. & McManus P. Responses to our critics. *BMJ*. 10 June 2003. https://www.bmj.com/content/326/7397/1008/rapid-responses (accessed 3 July 2020).

464   Hickie, I. *Curriculum vitae: Ian Hickie*. Sydney: Brain & Mind Research Institute. 23 August 2009. https://web.archive.org/web/20100331230312/http://www.bmri.org.au/about/Hickie_CV.pdf (accessed 3 December 2020).

465   'Pfizer Pharmaceuticals was involved not only as a program sponsor for 2002, but also provided a team of representatives to assist in the promotion, running, organising and recruiting of participants attending the Introductory Training Program. Pfizer also sponsored the running of train the trainer meetings in each state, and provided funding for the development of materials (CDROMs, workbooks etc). Pfizer had no input into the academic or educational content of any of the materials' Saegi, Tina, Forde, Blythe, & Duncan, Shane. (2003). *2002 annual activity report*. Box Hill, VIC: Educational Health Solutions. https://web.archive.org/web/20090930/http://www.spheregp.com.au/images/pdfs/SPHEREAnnualReport2002.pdf (accessed 10 December 2020).

466   Davies, Julie-Anne. GP jaunts 'boosted' drug sales. *The Australian*. 10 July 2010. https://www.theaustralian.com.au/news/health-science/gp-jaunts-boosted-drug-sales/news-story/37e3522ccf1453 3c143f32424d6109aa (accessed 10 December 2020).

467   Rosenberg, Sebastian, & Hickie, Ian. (2010, December). How to tackle a giant: creating a genuine evaluation of the Better Access Program. *Australasian Psychiatry*, 18(6), 496-502. https://journals.sagepub.com/doi/10.3109/10398562.2010.525642 (accessed 10 December 2020). (p. 501).

468   Cockayne, N. L., Duffy, S. L., Bonomally, R., English, A., Amminger, P. G., Mackinnon, A., Christensen, H. M., Naismith, S. L., & Hickie, I. B. (2015) The Beyond Ageing Project Phase 2 – a double-blind, selective prevention, randomised, placebo-controlled trial of omega-3 fatty acids and sertraline in an older age cohort at risk for depression: study protocol for a randomized controlled trial. *Trials*, *16*, 247. doi:10.1186/s13063-015-0762-6. https://trialsjournal.biomedcentral.com/articles/10.1186/s13063-015-0762-6 (15 August 2020).

469   Coupland CAC, et al. A study of the safety and harms of antidepressant drugs for older people: a cohort study using a large primary care database. National Institute for Health Research Health Technology Assessment programme: Executive Summaries https://www.ncbi.nlm.nih.gov/books/NBK63665/ (accessed 16 August 2020).

470   Hickie I. (2018). Curriculum Vitae: Ian Hickie AM MD FRANZCP FASSA. Available at: http://api.profiles.sydney.edu.au/AcademicProfiles/profile/resource?urlid=ian.hickie&type=cv (Accessed 18 November 2019).

471   Hickie, I. *Curriculum vitae: Ian Hickie*. Sydney: Brain & Mind Research Institute. 23 August 2009. https://web.archive.org/web/20100331230312/http://www.bmri.org.au/about/Hickie_CV.pdf (accessed 3 December 2020).

472   Cockayne, N. L., Duffy, S. L., Bonomally, R., English, A., Amminger, P. G., Mackinnon, A., Christensen, H. M., Naismith, S. L., & Hickie, I. B. (2015) The Beyond Ageing Project Phase 2 – a double-blind, selective prevention, randomised, placebo-controlled trial of omega-3 fatty acids and sertraline in an older age cohort at risk for depression: study protocol for a randomized controlled trial. *Trials*, *16*, 247. doi:10.1186/s13063-015-0762-6. https://trialsjournal.biomedcentral.com/articles/10.1186/s13063-015-0762-6 (accessed15 August 2020).

473   Coupland CAC, et al. A study of the safety and harms of antidepressant drugs for older people: a cohort study using a large primary care database. National Institute for Health Research Health Technology Assessment programme: Executive Summaries https://www.ncbi.nlm.nih.gov/books/NBK63665/ (accessed 16 August 2020).

474   Hickie I. Antidepressants in elderly people *BMJ*, 2 August 2011.

475   Hickie, I. (2011). Beyond Ageing Project: Phase 2 Participant Information Sheet. University of Sydney and Australian National University. Undated (created 25/06/2011, modified 24/10/2011)..

476   Meeter, M, Murre, J. M. J., Janssen, S. M. J., Birkenhager, T., & van den Broek, W. W. (2011). Retrograde amnesia after electroconvulsive therapy: A temporary effect? *Journal of Affective Disorders*, 132(1-2) 216–222. doi:10.1016/j.jad.2011.02.026. https://www.sciencedirect.com/science/article/pii/S0165032711000802 (accessed 27 July 2020).

477   Read J, & Bentall R (2010). The effectiveness of electroconvulsive therapy: a literature

review. *Epidemiologia e Psichiatria Sociale*, 19(4), 333-347. http://psychrights.org/Research/Digest/Electroshock/2010ReadBentallElectroshockReview.pdf (accessed 27 July 2020).

478   Gregory-Roberts, E. M., Naismith, S. L., Cullen, K. M., & Hickie, I. B. (2010). Electroconvulsive therapy-induced persistent retrograde amnesia: could it be minimised by ketamine or other pharmacological approaches? *Journal of Affective Disorders*, 126(1-2), 39-45. https://www.sciencedirect.com/science/article/abs/pii/S0165032709005254 (accessed 11 December 2020).

479   Gregory-Roberts, E. M., Naismith, S. L., Cullen, K. M., & Hickie, I. B. (2010). Electroconvulsive therapy-induced persistent retrograde amnesia: could it be minimised by ketamine or other pharmacological approaches? *Journal of Affective Disorders*, 126(1-2), 39-45. https://www.sciencedirect.com/science/article/abs/pii/S0165032709005254 (accessed 11 December 2020).

480   Read J, & Bentall R (2010). The effectiveness of electroconvulsive therapy: a literature review. *Epidemiologia e Psichiatria Sociale*, 19(4), 333-347. http://psychrights.org/Research/Digest/Electroshock/2010ReadBentallElectroshockReview.pdf (accessed 27 July 2020).

481   Stark, J (2010). Call for ban on shock therapy *The Age, December 19*. https://www.theage.com.au/national/victoria/call-for-ban-on-shock-therapy-20101218-191e2.html (accessed 5 December 2020)..

482   National Health and Medical Research Council (2015) NHMRC Research Achievements – Summary: All available end of grant reports as at 13 June 2014: outcomes of NHMRC funded research ending 2000 to 2013. Canberra: National Health and Medical Research Council. http://www.nhmrc.gov.au/grants-funding/research-funding-statistics-and-data/funding-statistics-outcomes-nhmrc-funded-researc (Accessed 22 January 2015).

483   National Health and Medical Research Council (2015) NHMRC Research Achievements – Summary: All available end of grant reports as at 13 June 2014: outcomes of NHMRC funded research ending 2000 to 2013. Canberra: National Health and Medical Research Council. http://www.nhmrc.gov.au/grants-funding/research-funding-statistics-and-data/funding-statistics-outcomes-nhmrc-funded-researc (Accessed 22 January 2015).

484   Hickie I. Lack of headspace data a hindrance Medical Observer. 8 April 2014 https://www.ausdoc.com.au/news/lack-headspace-data-hindrance (Accessed 5 December 2020)..

485   Stark J. Bitter rift on youth mental health provider headspace *Sydney Morning Herald* April 13, 2014 https://www.smh.com.au/national/bitter-rift-on-youth-mental-health-provider-headspace-20140412-36k60.html (Accessed 10 December 2020).

486   Hickie, Ian B. (2011). Antidepressants in elderly people. *BMJ*, 343:d4660 doi: 10.1136/*bmj.d4660*. https://www.*bmj*.com/content/343/*bmj*.d4660 (accessed 11 December 2020). (p. 2)..

487   Hickie, I. B., & Rogers, N. L. (2011). Novel melatonin-based therapies: Potential advances in the treatment of major depression. *Lancet*, 378(9791), 621-631. https://www.thelancet.com/journals/lancet/article/PIIS0140-6736(11)60095-0/fulltext (accessed 10 December 2020).

488   Hickie, I. B., & Rogers, N. L. (2011). Novel melatonin-based therapies: Potential advances in the treatment of major depression. *Lancet*, 378(9791), 621-631. https://www.thelancet.com/journals/lancet/article/PIIS0140-6736(11)60095-0/fulltext (10 December 2020).

489   *The Lancet*, 379(9812) https://www.thelancet.com/journals/lancet/issue/vol379no9812/PIIS0140-6736(12)X6003-3 (accessed 6 December 2020).

490   *The Lancet*, 379(9812) https://www.thelancet.com/journals/lancet/issue/vol379no9812/PIIS0140-6736(12)X6003-3 (accessed 6 December 2020).

491   Horton R. Twitter Account. 20-21 January 2012 http://twitter.com/richardhorton1 (accessed 22 January 2012).

492   Hickie, I. (2012). Ian Hickie: on Twitter, *The Lancet* and my critics. Crikey. 15 February 2012. https://www.crikey.com.au/2012/02/15/ian-hickie-responds-to-critics/ (accessed 22 July 2020).

493   Hickie, I. (2012). Ian Hickie: on Twitter, *The Lancet* and my critics. Crikey. 15 February 2012. https://www.crikey.com.au/2012/02/15/ian-hickie-responds-to-critics/ (accessed 22 July 2020).

494   Hickie, I. (2012). Ian Hickie: on Twitter, *The Lancet* and my critics. Crikey. 15 February 2012. https://www.crikey.com.au/2012/02/15/ian-hickie-responds-to-critics/ (accessed 22 July 2020).

495   Mayze, T. (2010). Servier Foundation Depression Masterclass Conference Review. November 2010 https://www.researchreview.com.au/au/clinical-area/psychiatry/psychiatry/servier-foundation-depression-masterclass-reviewed.aspx (20 July 2020). See also 1 Boring Old Man (2012) 'long overdue...' http://1boringoldman.com/index.php/2012/01/26/long-overdue/ (includes an image from Mayze (2010) that details Hickie's role).

496   Rose D. New antidepressant aims to restore internal body clock. *Medical Observer.* 11 Apr 2011. https://www.ausdoc.com.au/specialist-update/new-antidepressant-aims-restore-internal-body-clock (accessed 6 December 2020).

497   Naismith, S., Hermens, D., Bolitho, S., Ip, T., Scott, E., Rogers, N., Hickie, I. (2012), Circadian profiles in young people during the early stages of affective disorder. *Translational Psychiatry.* 2, e123. https://www.nature.com/articles/tp201247 (accessed 10 December 2020).

498   Corrigendum. *Translational Psychiatry* (2013) 3, e217; doi:10.1038/tp.2012.127. https://www. nature.com/articles/tp2012127 (accessed 10 December 2020).

499   Hickie I. Rogers N. Novel melatonin-based treatments for major depression – Authors' reply. *Lancet* January 21 https://www.the*lancet*.com/journals/*lancet*/article/PIIS0140-6736(12)60099-3/ fulltext (accessed 3 August 2020).

500   Hickie, I. (2012). Ian Hickie: on Twitter, *The Lancet* and my critics. Crikey. 15 February 2012. https://www.crikey.com.au/2012/02/15/ian-hickie-responds-to-critics/ (accessed 22 July 2020)..

501   Hickie I. Rogers N. Novel melatonin-based treatments for major depression – Authors' reply. *Lancet* January 21 https://www.the*lancet*.com/journals/*lancet*/article/PIIS0140-6736(12)60099-3/ fulltext (accessed 3 August 2020).

502   The Hon. Mark Butler MP, Leading Australians to Spearhead National Mental Health Reform (media release), 11 December 2011.

503   Dunlevy S. Campaign Targets Depression Guru, *The Australian,* Monday 13 February 2012. https://www.theaustralian.com.au/news/health-science/campaign-targets-depression-guru/news-stor y/14c29f9bc9778c409892417896ad08a6 (accessed 6 December 2020).

504   Hickie et al. Right care, first time: a highly personalised and measurement-based care model to manage youth mental health. *Medical Journal of Australia* 4 November 2019 https://www.mja.com.au/ journal/2019/211/9/right-care-first-time-highly-personalised-and-measurement-based-care-model (accessed 24 July 2020).

505   PricewaterhouseCoopers (2020). Using tech to support mental health treatment. https://www. pwc.com.au/about-us/solving-important-problems/using-tech-to-support-mental-health-treatment. html (accessed 15 August 2020).

506   Rosenberg S. Hickie I. Making better choices about mental health investment: The case for urgent reform of Australia's Better Access Program. *Australia and New Zealand Journal of Psychiatry* Volume: 53 issue: 11, November 1, 2019 p.1057 https://journals.sagepub.com/doi/ abs/10.1177/0004867419865335 (accessed 2 August 2020).

507   Rosenberg, S, Hickie, I, & Rock, D. (2020). Rethinking Mental Health in Australia: Adapting to the challenges of COVID-19 and planning for a brighter future. Sydney: Brain and Mind Centre. https://www.sydney.edu.au/content/dam/corporate/documents/brain-and-mind-centre/youthe/ rethinking-the-mental-health-of-australia.pdf (accessed 16 August 2020).

508   Meredith Griffiths Psychiatrist claims campaign to discredit him. ABC Radio The World Today. 13 Feb 2012 https://www.abc.net.au/radio/programs/worldtoday/psychiatrist-claims-campaign-to-discredit-him/3827172 (accessed 30 June 2020).

509   Ian Hickie: on Twitter, *The Lancet* and my critics. Crikey. 15 February 2012. https://www.crikey.com.au/2012/02/15/ian-hickie-responds-to-critics/ (accessed 22 July 2020).

510   Meredith Griffiths Psychiatrist claims campaign to discredit him. ABC Radio The World Today. 13 Feb 2012 https://www.abc.net.au/radio/programs/worldtoday/psychiatrist-claims-campaign-to-discredit-him/3827172 (accessed 30 June 2020).

511   ABC mental health initiative Mental As hits fundraising target with over $1m donated to research. ABC News Online. 11 October 2014 https://www.abc.net.au/news/2014-10-11/donations-in-abc-mental-health-fundraiser-pass-1-million/5806630 (accessed 30 June 2020).

512   Mental Health Australia CEO's Weekly Update - 15 August 2014 https://mhaustralia.org/ newsletters-bulletins/mhca-ceos-weekly-update-15-august (accessed 30 June 2020).

513   Mental Health Australia Website previously available at http://mhaustralia.org/about-us/ pharma-collaboration (accessed 30 July 2019).

514   Whitely M (2011) Hansard Western Australian Parliament [Wednesday, 25 May 2011] pp. 3984d-3994a. http://www.parliament.wa.gov.au/Hansard/hansard. nsf/0/75032653ddacbe7f482578b100299ab4/$FILE/A38+S1+20110525+p3984d-3994a.pdf (accessed 11 February 2019).

515   Peter Gøtzsche, Deadly Psychiatry and Organised Denial. People's Press 2015.

516   National Mental Health Commission, 2014: The National Review of Mental Health Programmes and Services. Sydney: NMHC Published by: National Mental Health Commission, Sydney.

517   https://www.abc.net.au/7.30/secret-report-reveals-disturbing-information-about/6392922.

518   Andy Park, Managing the maze of child mental health. ABC *7.30 Report* Posted Thu 20 Jun 2019, 8:25pm https://www.abc.net.au/7.30/managing-the-maze-of-child-mental-health/11233036 (accessed 2 July 2020).

519   Timmins P. Drug secrecy law trumps FOI. The Privacy Blogspot. 1 June 2010 http://foi-privacy.blogspot.com/2010/06/drug-secrecy-law-trumps-foi.html#.XIj0xSIzbIU (accessed 21 June 2020).

520   Administrative Appeals Tribunal of Australia Website. Whitely and Department of Health and Ageing [2010] AATA 338 (7 May 2010) http://www8.austlii.edu.au/cgi-bin/viewdoc/au/cases/cth/AATA/2010/338.html (accessed 14 March 2019).

521   Timmins P. Blog - Drug secrecy law trumps FOI. 1 June 2010. Available at http://foi-privacy.blogspot.com/2010/06/drug-secrecy-law-trumps-foi.html#.XIj0xSIzbIU (accessed 14 March 2019).

522   Adverse Drug Reactions Advisory Committee (Therapeutic Goods Administration). Suicidality with SSRIs: adults and children. Australian Adverse Drug Reactions Bulletin (August 2005) 24(5). Available at: https://www.tga.gov.au/publication-issue/australian-adverse-drug-reactions-bulletin-vol-24-no-4#a1 (Accessed 19 November 2019).

523   Australian Government. Therapeutic Goods Amendment (Repeal of Ministerial Responsibility for Approval of RU486) Bill 2005. Community Affairs Legislation Committee (3 February 2006).

524   M Rout, "Vioxx maker Merck and Co drew up doctor hit list" *The Australian* 1 April 2009. https://www.news.com.au/news/drug-company-drew-up-doctor-hit-list/news-story/eb55ca36e081d497730629e6c8559abf?sv=1f029b17d33bdbde184dbc4c4fed7126 (accessed 14 March 2019).

525   Sophie Scott and Alison Branley, 'Makers of blood-thinning drug Pradaxa "put marketing ahead of safety", British Medical Journal finds', ABC News, 4 August 2014. https://www.abc.net.au/news/2014-08-04/study-finds-information-on-anti-clotting-drug-pradaxa-withheld/5642436 (accessed 21 June 2020).

526   Quentin McDermott and Karen Michelmore, Patients Reveal Agony of Toxic Hip Implants, ABC Online Updated 16 May 2011, 9:20am http://www.abc.net.au/news/2011-05-16/patients-reveal-agony-of-toxic-hip-implants/2694656 (accessed 14 March 2019).

527   Sophie Scott and Alison Branley, Pelvic mesh implants 'one of the biggest medical scandals' involving Australian women. ABC News. Updated 28 Mar 2018. Available at https://www.abc.net.au/news/2018-03-28/pelvic-mesh-implants-only-used-as-last-resort-senate-report/9592384 (accessed 14 March 2019).

528   Australian Government Response to Senate Community Affairs References Committee Report on The role of the Therapeutic Goods Administration regarding medical devices, particularly Poly Implant Prothèse (PIP) breast implants. July 2013. https://www.health.gov.au/internet/main/publishing.nsf/Content/B1ABE3987E9644F6CA257BF0001A34D9/$File/PIP%20breast%20implants.pdf (accessed 14 March 2019).

529   Joseph S. Ross et al, 'Guest Authorship and Ghostwriting in Publications Related to Rofecoxib: A Case Study of Industry Documents from Rofecoxib Litigation', *Journal of American Medical Association*, 299: 15 2008.

530   M Rout, 'Vioxx maker Merck and Co drew up doctor hit list'. *The Australian*. 1 April 2009. https://www.news.com.au/news/drug-company-drew-up-doctor-hit-list/news-story/eb55ca36e081d497730629e6c8559abf?sv=1f029b17d33bdbde184dbc4c4fed7126 (accessed 14 March 2019).

531   Vioxx was an arthritis and acute pain medication that was launched in the United States in 1999 by Merck & Co and was marketed in over eighty countries. Sales in 2003 were worth $2.5 billion. In March 2000 the results of a study, the Vioxx Gastrointestinal Outcomes Research (VIGOR), indicated an increased risk of cardiovascular events. This trial found that there was an increased relative risk for confirmed cardiovascular events, such as heart attack and stroke, 18 months after treatment began. 'Merck Announces Voluntary Worldwide Withdrawal of VIOXX®', available at http://www.merck.com/newsroom/vioxx/pdf/vioxx_press_release_final.pdf (accessed 7 February 2007). Merck failed to

warn treating doctors or patients about the results of the VIGOR study (2000). No information, let alone warnings, about the risks were given, until some two years later. Even then the information that was finally given was unclear. Consequently, doctors and patients continued prescribing and using Vioxx until its withdrawal. As a result, thousands of people may have suffered serious injury or died as a result.

532   Deborah Cohen, 'Dabigatran: how the drug company withheld important analyses', *BMJ, 349, g4670, July 2014*. Available at http://www.*bmj*.com/content/349/*bmj*.g4670 (accessed 21 June 2020).

533   Sophie Scott and Alison Branley, 'Makers of blood-thinning drug Pradaxa "put marketing ahead of safety", British Medical Journal finds', ABC News, 4 August 2014. https://www.abc.net.au/news/2014-08-04/study-finds-information-on-anti-clotting-drug-pradaxa-withheld/5642436 (accessed 21 June 2020).

534   Sophie Scott and Alison Branley, 'Makers of blood-thinning drug Pradaxa "put marketing ahead of safety", British Medical Journal finds', ABC News, 4 August 2014. https://www.abc.net.au/news/2014-08-04/study-finds-information-on-anti-clotting-drug-pradaxa-withheld/5642436 (accessed 21 June 2020).

535   Deborah Cohen, 'Dabigatran: how the drug company withheld important analyses', *BMJ, 349, g4670, July 2014*. Available at http://www.*bmj*.com/content/349/*bmj*.g4670 (accessed 21 June 2020).

536   A federal judge in Illinois, overseeing a court case concerning whether consumers were warned by the manufacturer of Pradaxa about the risks, released internal emails, memos and internal presentations which related to whether an upcoming research paper would impact on the main selling point of Pradaxa. Katie Thomas, 'Study of Drug for Blood Clots Caused a Stir, Records Show', *New York Times*, 5 February 2014. http://www.nytimes.com/2014/02/06/business/study-of-blood-clot-drug-pradaxa-unnerved-its-maker-documents-suggest.html (accessed 21 June 2020).

537   Katie Thomas, 'Study of Drug for Blood Clots Caused a Stir, Records Show', *The New York Times*, 5 February 2014. Available at http://www.nytimes.com/2014/02/06/business/study-of-blood-clot-drug-pradaxa-unnerved-its-maker-documents-suggest.html (accessed 21 June 2020).

538   Sophie Scott and Alison Branley, 'Makers of blood-thinning drug Pradaxa "put marketing ahead of safety", British Medical Journal finds', ABC News, 4 August 2014. https://www.abc.net.au/news/2014-08-04/study-finds-information-on-anti-clotting-drug-pradaxa-withheld/5642436 (accessed 21 June 2020).

539   Paul A. Reilly, et al, 'The Effect of Dabigatran Plasma Concentrations and Patient Characteristics on the Frequency of Ischemic Stroke and Major Bleeding in Atrial Fibrillation Patients: The RE-LY Trial (Randomized Evaluation of Long-Term Anticoagulation Therapy)', *Journal of the American College of Cardiology*, Vol. 63, Issue 4, (2014), pp. 321-328.

540   Katie Thomas, 'Study of Drug for Blood Clots Caused a Stir, Records Show', *The New York Times*, 5 February 2014. Available at http://www.nytimes.com/2014/02/06/business/study-of-blood-clot-drug-pradaxa-unnewarved-its-maker-documents-suggest.html (accessed 21 June 2020).

541   Husten L. Boehringer Ingelheim Settles US Pradaxa Litigation For $650 Million. *Forbes*. https://www.*forbes*.com/sites/larryhusten/2014/05/28/boehringer-ingelheim-settles-us-pradaxa-litigation-for-650-million/#6d8d53d42ae6 (accessed 23 May 2020).

542   Allen Frances, M.D. *Saving Normal: An Insider's Revolt against Out-of-Control Psychiatric Diagnosis, DSM-5, Big Pharma, and the Medicalization of Ordinary Life*, HarperCollins, New York 2013, p.96.

543   Horton Richard (editorial), Lawsuits alone will not fix the US opioid overdose crisis. *The Lancet*. 7 September 2019. https://www.the*lancet*.com/journals/*lancet*/article/PIIS0140-6736(19)32041-0/fulltext (accessed 22 June 2020).

544   Gelineau K. Opioid crisis goes global as deaths surge in Australia AP News. September 6, 2019. https://apnews.com/cfc86f47e03843849a89ab3fce44c73c (accessed 22 June 2020)..

545   G. Chouinard, L. Annable, and J. Bradwejn, 'An early phase II clinical trial of tomoxetine (LY139603) in the treatment of newly admitted depressed patients', Psychopharmacology 1984, 83, p.126.

546   Wietecha L. et al. Atomoxetine Increased Effect over Time in Adults with Attention-Deficit/Hyperactivity Disorder Treated for up to 6 Months: Pooled Analysis of Two Double-Blind, Placebo-Controlled, Randomized Trials. CNS Neuroscience Therapeutics. July 2016. https://www.ncbi.nlm.nih.gov/pmc/articles/PMC5069588/ (accessed 22 June 2020).

547   U.S. Food and Drug Administration. 'New Warning for Strattera' *Science Daily*, 22 December 2004. www.sciencedaily.com/releases/2004/12/041219133156.htm (accessed 22 June 2020).

548   U.S. Food and Drug Administration. Public health advisory: Suicidal thinking in children and adolescents being treated with Strattera (atomoxetine). 29 September 2005. http://www.fda.gov/cder/drug/advisory/atomoxetine.htm (accessed 22 June 2020).

549   Australian Government Department of Health Therapeutic goods Administration. Atomoxetine (Straterra) - risk of increased blood pressure and/or heart rate. http://www.tga.gov.au/safety/alerts-medicine-atomoxetine-111102.htm (accessed 22 June 2020).

550   A 2008 study by Curtin University pharmacologist Con Berbatis identified that only a tiny fraction (for general practitioners in Australia only 2 per cent) of adverse events are reported. Con Berbatis, 'Primary care and Pharmacy: 4. Large contributions to national adverse reaction reporting by pharmacists in Australia', *i2P E-Magazine*, Issue 72, June 2008, p. 1.

551   Adverse events information related to Strattera obtained from the Therapeutic Goods Administration's Public Case Detail reports.

552   Australian Government Department of Health Therapeutic goods Administration. Atomoxetine and suicidality in children and adolescents. https://www.tga.gov.au/publication-issue/medicines-safety-update-volume-4-number-5-october-2013#atomoxetine (accessed 22 June 2020).

553   A 2008 study by Curtin University pharmacologist Con Berbatis identified that for the prescription of all drugs by Australian General Practitioners only two percent of adverse events are reported to the TGA. Con Berbatis (2008), 'Primary care and Pharmacy: 4. Large contributions to national adverse reaction reporting by pharmacists in Australia', *i2P E-Magazine*, Issue 72, June 2008..

554   Watson M. Deep sleep therapy and Chelmsford Private Hospital: have we learnt anything? *Australasian Psychiatry* 21(3):206-212 June 2013 file:///C:/Users/177421E/Downloads/deepsleeparticle.pdf.

555   Olfson M, Marcus SC. National trends in outpatient psychotherapy. *American Journal of Psychiatry*. December 2010 pp.1456-63. https://pubmed.ncbi.nlm.nih.gov/20686187/ (accessed 22 June 2020).

556   Harris G. Talk doesn't pay, so psychiatry turns to drug therapy. *The New York Times*. 2011 Mar 5 [cited 2011 Mar 6]. Available from: http://www.nytimes.com/2011/03/06/health/policy/06doctors.html (accessed 22 June 2020).

557   Goetze P. Does long term use of psychiatric drugs cause more harm than good? Yes. *BMJ*. 12 May 2015 https://www.*bmj*.com/content/350/*bmj*.h2435.full (accessed 22 June 2020).

558   GlaxoSmithKline, *Prescribing Information – Dexedrine (dextroamphetamine sulphate)*. https://www.accessdata.fda.gov/drugsatfda_docs/label/2007/017078s042lbl.pdf (accessed 22 June 2020) And Ritalin Prescribing Information https://www.accessdata.fda.gov/drugsatfda_docs/label/2013/010187s077lbl.pdf (accessed 22 June 2020).

559   Timothy E. Wilens Impact of ADHD and Its Treatment on Substance Abuse in Adults, *Journal of Clinical Psychiatry*, 2004 http://www.izun.org.il/imageBank/articales/2004.pdf (accessed 22 June 2020).

560   Moynihan R. Cassels A. *Selling Sickness*, Allen and Unwin 2005. pp. 66–67.

561   Hall T. Shifting the focus of the mental health system. ABC The Drum: Opinion. 14 April 2011.

562   Whiteford HA, Meurk C, Carstensen G, Hall W, Hill P, Head BW. How did youth mental health make it onto Australia's 2011 federal policy agenda? SAGE Open 2016. https://journals.sagepub.com/doi/pdf/10.1177/2158244016680855 (accessed 22 June 2020).

563   Term of reference for the Royal Commission available at https://s3.ap-southeast-2.amazonaws.com/hdp.au.prod.app.vic-rcvmhs.files/3515/6764/2426/Terms_of_Reference_signed.pdf (accessed 22 June 2020).

564   Whitely M. Hansard West Australian Legislative Assembly. Wednesday, 30 November 2011. p10216b-10230a. Available at https://www.parliament.wa.gov.au/Hansard%5Chansard.nsf/0/39ae17f1980cf5094825795a0031f6fc/$FILE/A38%20S1%2020111130%20p10216b-10230a.pdf (accessed 22 June 2020).

565   *The Australian* Institute of Health and Welfare (AIHW) estimates that spending on mental health-related services in Australia from all sources (government and non-government) was around $9.0 billion, or $373 per person, in 2015–16. Of the $9.0 billion, $5.4 billion (59.8%) was funded by

state and territory governments, $3.1 billion (35.0%) was funded by *the Australian* Government, and $466 million (5.2%) was funded by private health insurance funds.In 2016–17, *the Australian* Government spent: $1.2 billion on Medicare-subsidised mental health-specific services ($49 per person) and $511 million on mental health-related subsidised prescriptions under the Pharmaceutical Benefits Scheme (PBS) and the Repatriation Pharmaceutical Benefits Scheme (RPBS) ($21 per person). https://www.aph.gov.au/About_Parliament/Parliamentary_Departments/Parliamentary_Library/pubs/rp/rp1819/Quick_Guides/MentalHealth (accessed 22 June 2020).

566   Whitely MP. Attention Deficit Hyperactivity Disorder Policy, Practice and Regulatory Capture in Australia 1992–2012 [PhD]. Perth, WA: Curtin University; 2014. https://espace.curtin.edu.au/bitstream/handle/20.500.11937/1776/225953_Whitely%202014.pdf?sequence=2&isAllowed=y (accessed 15 June 2020).

567   House of Commons Health Committee (2005), The Influence of the Pharmaceutical Industry: Fourth Report of Session 2004-05, Vol. 1, London, The Stationery Office, pp.97-109. Available at http://www.publications.parliament.uk/pa/cm200405/cmselect/cmhealth/42/42.pdf (accessed 23 May 2013).

568   House of Commons Health Committee (2005), The Influence of the Pharmaceutical Industry: Fourth Report of Session 2004-05, Vol. 1, London, The Stationery Office, pp.97-109. http://www.publications.parliament.uk/pa/cm200405/cmselect/cmhealth/42/42.pdf (accessed 23 May 2013). .

569   House of Commons Health Committee (2005), The Influence of the Pharmaceutical Industry: Fourth Report of Session 2004-05, Vol. 1, London, The Stationery Office, p.102 http://www.publications.parliament.uk/pa/cm200405/cmselect/cmhealth/42/42.pdf (accessed 23 May 2013). .

570   Tara John, How the World's First Loneliness Minister Will Tackle 'the Sad Reality of Modern Life'. Time, 25 April 2018. http://time.com/5248016/tracey-crouch-uk-loneliness-minister/ (accessed 15 April 2019).

571   Lee Mannion, Britain appoints minister for loneliness amid growing isolation. Reuters, 17 January 2018. https://www.reuters.com/article/us-britain-politics-health/britain-appoints-minister-for-loneliness-amid-growing-isolation-idUSKBN1F61I6 (accessed 15 April 2019).

572   UK Office of National Statistics Website. Loneliness —What characteristics and circumstances are associated with feeling lonely? Which factors independently affect loneliness? https://www.ons.gov.uk/peoplepopulationandcommunity/wellbeing/articles/lonelinesswhatcharacteristicsandcircumstancesareassociatedwithfeelinglonely/2018-04-10#which-factors-independently-affect-loneliness (accessed 15 April 2019).

573   Entis L. Scientists are working on a pill for loneliness, *The Guardian Australia*. 26 January 2019. https://www.theguardian.com/us-news/2019/jan/26/pill-for-loneliness-psychology-science-medicine?fbclid=IwAR1RbNnmZojZSI7i6xFI1DbuPoTmcB2Qd2azFR-Lhlc8q9S8pK7zXnJGooU (accessed 15 April 2019).